Alkaline Vegan Drinks
Have More Energy, Lose Weight and Stimulate Massive Healing!

Over 140 Recipes Including Teas, Smoothies & Juices
Vegan-Paleo and Alkaline Approved

By Karen Greenvang
Copyright ©Karen Greenvang 2016

All rights reserved. No part of this publication may be reproduced, stored in a retrieval system, or transmitted, in any form or by any means, electronic, mechanical, photocopying, recording or otherwise, without the prior written permission of the author and the publishers.

Free Complimentary eBook Available At:

www.holisticwellnessbooks.com/vegan

The scanning, uploading, and distribution of this book via the Internet, or via any other means, without the permission of the author is illegal and punishable by law. Please purchase only authorized electronic editions, and do not participate in or encourage electronic piracy of copyrighted materials.

All information in this book has been carefully researched and checked for factual accuracy. However, the author and publishers make no warranty, expressed or implied, that the information contained herein is appropriate for every individual, situation or purpose, and assume no responsibility for errors or omission. The reader assumes the risk and full responsibility for all actions, and the author will not be held liable for any loss or damage, whether consequential, incidental, and special or otherwise, that may result from the information presented in this publication.

All cooking is an experiment in a sense, and many people come to the same or similar recipe over time. All recipes in this book have been derived from author's personal experience. Should any bear a close resemblance to those used elsewhere, that is purely coincidental.

The book is not intended to provide medical advice or to take the place of medical advice and treatment from your personal physician. Readers are advised to consult their own doctors or other qualified health professionals regarding the treatment of medical conditions. The author shall not be held liable or responsible for any misunderstanding or misuse of the information contained in this book. The information is not intended to diagnose, treat or cure any disease.

It is important to remember that the author of this book is not a doctor/ medical professional. Only opinions based upon her own personal experiences or research are cited. THE AUTHOR DOES NOT OFFER MEDICAL ADVICE or prescribe any treatments. For any health or medical issues – you should be talking to your doctor first.

Contents

INTRODUCTION 7

TIPS ON CREATING THE PERFECT DRINKS 11

RECIPE MEASUREMENTS 12

SMOOTHIES 13

    A TROPICAL MORNING 15
    RASPBERRY AND ORANGE POWER BLEND 16
    ORCHARD IN A GLASS 17
    BANANA BAKEWELL TART 18
    GREEN GODDESS 19
    FRY UP 20
    LEFT OVERS SMOOTHIE 21
    THIA ME UP 22
    AN ENGLISH PICNIC 23
    CHESTNUTS ROASTING 24
    CHERRY, LIME AND COCONUT 25
    THIS LITTLE GREEN PIGGY 26
    PUMPKIN PIE SKINNY SMOOTHIE 27
    RASPBERRY CREAM PROTEIN SMOOTHIE 28
    BRUSSEL MUSCLE 29
    POWER PUNCH 30
    MY KIWI COFFEE 31
    A SUGAR FIX 32
    DARK CHOCOLATE "MILK SHAKE" 33
    NUTTYLICIOUS 34
    TUTTI FRUITIE 35
    SWEET PASSION 36
    SESAME, BANANA AND COCONUT SLUSH 37
    VEGETABLE PIE 38
    FISH CAKE SMOOTHIE 39
    GOOD WEED 40
    TOFFEE APPLE SMOOTHIE 41
    LATE SUMMER SMOOTHIE 42
    RHUBARB AND CUSTARD 43
    KEY LIME SKINNY SMOOTHIE 44
    POWER TO THE PROTEIN 45
    POWER TO THE VANILLA PROTEIN! 46
    THE PURPLE BEAST 47
    RUBY RED 48

A French Summer 49
The Market Mix 50
Savory Notes 51
Skin Cream 52
Veggie Patch 53
Chest Health 54
Caca Maca 55
Anti-Inflammation 56
The Green Coco Bomb 57
The Speckled Egg 58
Peach On a Beach 59
The Energy Blend 60
Sweet Earth 61
Dragon Fire 62
Dragon Milk 63

JUICES 64

Refresher 67
Natures Pack Up 68
Sweet Earth 69
Cool As 70
Heat Me Up 71
Fruitful Fields 72
Great Scott 73
Strawberry Refresher 74
Where's The Orange? 75
Raspberry and Mango Punch 76
Hot Apple Shot 77
Italian Fashion 78
Green Queen 79
Vegging Out 80
Sweet and Sour 81
Chill On A Sunday 82
Fun Sun 83
Currant Brigade 84
"Corrr"dial Please 85
Kernel Colonel 86
Citron Whizz 87
Christmas Cheer 88
Boost To The Moon 89
Summer Sweetheart 90
Serene Dream 91
Traffic Lights 92
Turkish Delight 93

PLUM PUNCH 94
EASTERN LOVE 95
MELLOW YELLOW 96
HEAT SAUCE 97
MINT SHOT 98
A GOOD START 99
STRAWBERRY STARS 100
SWEETEST LEAF IN THE DRAWER 101
FRIENDLY MONSTER 102
FRIENDLY MONSTER MINI 103
HOT TOMATO 104
SUPER JUICE 105
TUMMY TREAT 106
PARSLEY PULSE 107
STRESS REDUCER 108

HERBAL INFUSIONS: TEAS AND TISANES 109

CINNAMON TEA 112
SLIPPERY ELM AND GINGER SETTLER 113
FENUGREEK, LIME LEAF AND TURMERIC TISANE 114
LEMON AND GINGER TONIC 115
NETTLE TEA 116
CUP MED 117
ARTICHOKE TEA 118
CARDAMOM AND VANILLA TEA 119
HERBAL FEAST TEA 120
ROSEMARY TEA 121
TURMERIC, LEMON AND GINGER BLEND 122
SLEEPY TURMERIC LATTE 123
TRANQUILLITY 124
BLACKCURRANT LEAF AND PEPPERMINT TEA 125
VANILLA, APRICOT AND MINT TEA 126
TURMERIC ORANGE SPLASH 127
FENNEL INFUSION 128
SAGE AND ONION "BROTH" 129
HIBISCUS BLEND 130
MINT TWIST 131
RASPBERRY AND MINT INFUSION 132
POPPY TONIC 133
LEMON AND TARRAGON BREW 134
SPICE BLEND 135
JUNIPER BERRY TEA 136
GINSENG GINGER TEA 137
VANILLA, ORANGE AND SAGE REMEDY 138

Elderberry and Cinnamon Tisane 139
Lavender Soother 140
Celery Seeds and Basil Cup 141
Parsley, Mint and Lemon Tisane 142
Green Tea and Tonic 143
A Noble Brew 144
A Bit About Infused Waters 145
Mint, Cucumber and Lime Vitality 147
Grapefruit and Rosemary Twining 148
Raspberry and Melon Infusion 149
Immune Booster 150
Detox Water 151
Passion Drink 152
Lemon, Ginger and Apple Infusion 153
Peach and Sage Herbal Hydration 154
Watermelon and Mint Refresher 155
Basil, Mint and Lemon Squeeze 156
Chia Strawberry Fruit Cup 157
Chia Mint Cup 158
Rose, Strawberry and Lemon Cooler 159
Cinnamon and Apple Water 160
Pomegranate, Lime and Ginger Infusion 162
Oregano, Blueberry and Lime Refresher 163
Coconut and Peach Infusion 164
Coconut Water Raspberry Lemon Mix 165
Pineapple and Mint Cup 166
Orange and Tarragon Refreshment 167
Thirst Quencher 168
Hibiscus, Lemon and Cherry Sour 169
Pink Lemon Aid 170

CONCLUSION 172

MORE BOOKS BY KAREN GREENVANG .... ERROR! BOOKMARK NOT DEFINED.

Introduction

Alkaline Vegan Drinks, aka Hydro-fitness is a book totally dedicated to get your body working at its best, through what you drink. It's a fantastic collection of inspirational, fun and tasty smoothies, juices and herbal teas and infusions that are great for your hydration and health. They are also paleo and vegan friendly. Perfect to alkalize your body and feel amazing! With carefully chosen spices and super foods to add some wonderful flavors and health benefits, this will be a regular book in the kitchen.

Dehydration can impact us all at times, whether in a mild or severe form. But there are ways to protect us from this and the symptoms and problems this can cause. Dizziness and light-headedness, headaches, tiredness, dry mouth and passing urine less than 3-4 times a day: These symptoms are troublesome and long term, extremely bad for our wellbeing.

We spend much more time than ever, keeping fit, ating better and being much more aware of medical conditions caused by our lifestyle, but why does hydration still get forgotten so easily? How many times have you got to the end of the day and thought; "Oh, I forgot to drink today!"? Being adequately hydrated will make you perform better, think better and feel better, so it is certainly one to be focused on.

Whilst we may forget to take in sufficient liquids during the day, it is likely this isn't also the case with the intake of coffee. Some of us can relate to the routine of dragging ourselves to the coffee machine in the morning, desperate for caffeine, so this isn't likely to be a forgotten drink! There are claims to suggest caffeine is a good addition to our diet and yes, Paleo foods do also include the word "coffee" on the list. However, abusing caffeine will certainly undo all the good things going on in your body with a healthy eating plan.

Alkaline Vegan Drinks aka Hydro Fitness will be providing you with a number of morning "pick me ups", that can replace the caffeine. You will be surprised how much better you will feel once your body has accepted that caffeine is no longer part of your diet and how much less work it will be doing to process this through your system. Symptoms such as headaches, insomnia, nausea, chest pains and palpitations are all avoidable when eradicating caffeine from your diet, especially when there are some great super foods that can still give you that get up and go.

So, how about we have some fun with drinks and give them as much thought as what you are going to eat for a dinner? The Vegan Paleo diet is rich with flavours that are a joy to eat and with some imagination, this can transform your drinking to something that will never be forgotten again!

Nature has so many wonderful ingredients to offer that are packed full of goodness. They can provide you with such stamina and vitality, so don't just eat them, add them to drinks too! Get energized and feel hydro-fit!

Before we get into it, I would like to offer you free access to my VIP newsletter. Through that newsletter, you will receive many bonuses, recipes , motivation and you will be notified about my new books at discounted prices. Oh, there will also be many giveaways that are exclusive to my subscribers. As a bonus, you will receive a bonus- free eBook with vegan smoothie recipes.

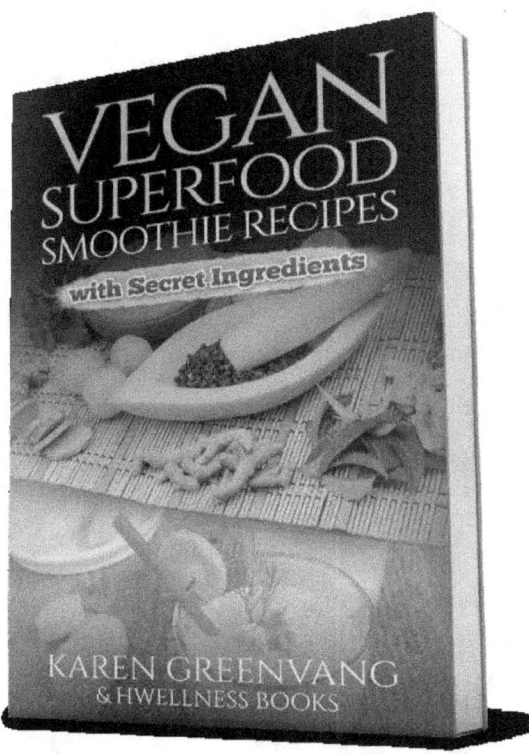

Simply visit:

www.holisticwellnessbooks.com/vegan to join my VIP email newsletter and grab your free copy now.

In case you happen to have any technical problems- email me at:

karen@holisticwellnessbooks.com and I will be happy to help!

Tips On Creating The Perfect Drinks

Ensure all of the ingredients you use are at their freshest. It would be a real shame to go to all the effort of planning on improving your hydration through these great recipes when the ingredients are lacking in their full available nutritional benefits.

Try and choose smoothies, juices or infusions that use seasonal ingredients. This ensures the produce you use is at it's best and will give the best flavor. Plus, seasonal fruit and vegetables do tend to cost a little less.

Try and chill glasses and serving items, before creating a cold smoothie, juice or infusion. This will keep your finished drink at an icy temperature for longer and will give the most refreshing experience.

Use the smoothies and juices pretty soon after making them. Each drink will begin to lose its nutritional value as it stands.

Recipe Measurements

I love keeping ingredient measurements as simple as possible- this is why I stick to tablespoons, teaspoons and cups.

The cup measurement I use is the American cup measurement. I also use it for dry ingredients. If you are new to it, let me help you:

If you don't have American Cup measures, just use a metric or imperial liquid measuring jug and fill your jug with your ingredient to the corresponding level. Here's how to go about it:

1 American Cup= 250ml= 8 fl.oz

For example:

If a recipe calls for 1 cup of almonds, simply place your almonds into your measuring jug until it reaches the 250 ml/8oz mark.

I know that different countries use different measurements and I wanted to make things simple for you.

Smoothies

It's worth a noting a few things about smoothies, before we run and get our blenders. Smoothies are different to Juices and there is a place in our lives for both.

Smoothies are made from "whole" ingredients. This means nothing is taken away. They are made in a high speed blender, which pulverizes the entire contents in to a smooth textured drink. Other items can be added to smoothies that aren't quite as successful in a Juicer – have you tried juicing an avocado before? Nut butters, seeds, oils, mushrooms and many, many more, are all examples of what can be blended in a smoothie, that need to stay out of the juicer!

The benefits of a smoothie include-
- You get the whole ingredient and therefore a much more nutrient dense drink, full of all the vitamins and minerals available.
- You get to include ingredients that you can't juice and still incorporate them in to a drink.
- They can feel a little more indulgent than a juice, even though they are still healthy!
- They will fill you up, as the insoluble fiber has not been removed.
- They also still contain soluble fiber that is associated with regulating blood sugar levels and lowering cholesterol.

- You can tailor them to meet your dietary requirements. For example, if you want a mood boosting drink, you can add Brazil nuts and their ability to create brain happy serotonin! Not getting adequate Omega 3? The produce a smoothie using Omega 3 rich seeds, like flax.
- Blenders are cheap to buy so an easy Hydro Fitness plan to begin with.
- Blenders are usually easy to clean.

The Not So Good Benefits
- It can be easy to over eat with smoothies. They can be used as a meal replacement or snack but ought not be to added to an already nutrition packed meal.

If you don't have a blender yet, don't despair. You may have a stick blender that you can try some of these recipes out on? So get whizzing and get drinking.

NOTE : All of these recipes serve 1-2 (depending if using it for a snack/meal)

A Tropical Morning

How about some sunshine in a glass to get you up in the morning? Pineapple is certainly a great flavor to get you energized first thing and is great stomach settler if it's been a long night.

Ingredients
- 1 small ripe banana
- 1 cup pineapple chunks
- 1 cup coconut milk

Instructions

1. Ensure the ingredients are all really cold before blending. You can use frozen bananas* for this recipe and this will add a really refreshing slushiness to it!

2. Chop the banana, if using a fresh one, and add to the blender with the pineapple and coconut milk.

3. Decorate with toasted coconut flakes if liked.

*Tip. Freeze bags of chopped bananas and take out handfuls for the base of all banana smoothies as they make a lovely icy drink without adding any more liquid in the form of ice cubes.

Raspberry and Orange Power Blend

These flavors work so well together and provide a gentle release of energy. Try and keep oranges you are going to juice at room temperature as they provide much more juice when they aren't fridge cold. The rest of the ingredients can be fridge cold.

Ingredients
- ½ cup goji berries
- ½ small banana
- 1 cup of raspberries
- 1 orange, juice only
- Extra Water to thin the smoothie, if you like

Instructions
1. Blend the goji berries on their own first, to try and produce a fine powder.

2. Add the raspberries, banana and orange juice and blend until smooth.

3. Add ice cubes or extra water as required.

Orchard In A Glass

This is a lovely sweet smoothie, all from natural sources with no added sweetener needed. The red apple provides even more sweetness, but you could opt for a sharper green one if you like.

Ingredients
- 13 oz can of pears in own juice (not syrup), drained
- 1 red apple
- 1 cup apple juice
- ½ cup almond milk (unsweetened)

Instructions
1. Put the pears in the blender.

2. Peel and core the apple and chop in to pieces and add to the blender too. Add the liquids and blend until smooth.

3. Add some ice and thin apple slices (rubbed with lemon) for decoration.

Banana Bakewell Tart

What a combination of flavors and a great twist on an old English Pudding. The ground almonds are added for the "pastry bottom", the raspberries for the jam and the almond butter for the buttery almond flavor. Yum!

Ingredients
- 1 ripe banana (frozen if liked)
- 1 cup almond milk, unsweetened
- 1 tsp ground almonds
- 1 tsp fresh raspberries
- 2 tbsp smooth almond butter
- 1 tsp toasted almonds

Instructions
1. Put the banana, milk, ground almonds and almond butter in to the blender and blend until really smooth.

2. Pour in to a cold glass* and serve sprinkled with the almonds

*Tip – Freeze your glass before serving (check it's freezer proof!) as it can keep a smoothie ice cold for longer.

Green Goddess

If it's green it MUST be good for you? How can it taste so good too though? Hemp has been added here to give you a real boost of energy. Be sure to use the shelled variety though or you will find the smoothie will never be smooth! This would make a great breakfast and has a little bit of sweetness from the pear.

Ingredients
- ½ avocado
- 1 cup coconut milk
- 4 cubes frozen spinach
- 1 pear
- 1 tsp hemp seeds, hulled (plus extra to sprinkle)

Instructions
1. Scoop out the avocado and add to a blender. Add the spinach.

2. Cut the pear in to slices, discarding the core. Add the hemp seeds and milk and blend well.

3. Serve with a sprinkling of hemp on top.

Fry Up

Need something savory first thing? We don't always want a massive hit of sweetness from a smoothie, so maybe try this as an alternative to a Paleo fry up?

Ingredients
- 4 cubes of frozen spinach
- ½ avocado
- 1 tsp nutritional yeast
- 1 tbsp cashew nuts
- 1 cup tomato juice
- 1 lime, juice
- Pinch of salt

Instructions
1. Place all the ingredients in to a blender and prepared to be surprised.

2. Serve in ice cold glasses.

Left Overs Smoothie

There always seems to be apples and oranges kicking about in the fruit bowl, so don't let them perish. Liven them up with some great added flavors and great hydration for the day

Ingredients
- 1 apple
- 1 orange
- 1 inch piece of root ginger
- ½ tsp turmeric
- 1 cup coconut water

Instructions
1. Peel the apple, remove the core and chop in to pieces. Add to the blender.

2. Peel the orange and remove the segments, add to the blender too.

3. Peel the ginger and add to the blender with the turmeric and coconut water.

4. Serve in an ice cold glass with ice cubes.

Thia Me Up

Lychees are a great fruit to add to your diet. They are full of Vitamin C, Vitamin B6, niacin and folate. They also have shown to have anti-viral properties and can help work against the herpes virus. They are lovely and sweet and a tasty addition to a smoothie.

Ingredients
- Handful of kale, tough stalks removed
- 6 Thai basil leaves
- 1 small apple
- 5 fresh lychees, peeled and stoned
- 1 cm fresh ginger root, roughly peeled
- ½ lime juice
- ½ cup of filtered water – more to mix if you like

Instructions
1. Place all of the ingredients in to a blender
2. Blend until smooth
3. Drink immediately, packed with ice.

An English Picnic

This recipe has a warming mix of mustard and apples. Added to by a healthy spoonful of walnuts and a refreshing lettuce, you just need a picnic blanket!

Ingredients
- 1 apple
- ½ small green lettuce
- 1 salad onion
- Small bunch of parsley
- ½ tsp yellow mustard
- 1 tsp walnut pieces
- 1 cup apple juice

Instructions
1. Add all of the ingredients in to a blender.

2. Blend until smooth and enjoy ice cold.

Chestnuts Roasting

This is a warming smoothie, served cold and full of chestnuts. Packed with Vitamin B6, potassium and copper, they are good to add to your diet, plus if you're watching your weight, these nuts are lower in fat and calories than other nuts. The maca, cacao and cinnamon add a toasty flavor of comfort.

Ingredients
- 1 cup of chestnuts, cooked and peeled
- 1 cup almond milk
- 1 tsp maca powder
- 1 tsp raw cacao powder
- ½ tsp cinnamon
- handful of ice

Instructions
1. Place all of the ingredients in to the blender
2. Blend until smooth.

Cherry, Lime and Coconut

Cherries are full of anti-oxidants. They have been associated with helping insomnia, reducing fat around the stomach area and also joint pain. They are so sweet and when added to by the sharp lime and soothing coconut, a healthy, perfectly balanced smoothie is created!

Ingredients
- 1 cup of ripe cherries, the darker the better
- 1 lime, juice only
- 1 cup coconut milk
- ½ banana, frozen

Instructions
1. Remove the stones from the cherries and juice the lime.
2. Add these and the other ingredients to a blender and blend until smooth.

This Little Green Piggy

Chlorophyll powder is becoming more and more popular when creating juices and smoothies. This pigment is known for promoting good health. The powder also claims it can control hunger, reduce body odor and encourage healing. It's really worth adding a variety of ingredients in to juices and smoothies as it's the best way for nature to provide you a whole array of nutrients.

Ingredients
- 1 handful of baby spinach leaves
- 1.5 inch barrel of cucumber
- 8 leaves fresh mint
- 1 cup of coconut milk
- 1 tsp chlorophyll powder
- Handful of ice

Instructions
1. Place all of the ingredients in to a blender

2. Blend until smooth and enjoy immediately.

Pumpkin Pie Skinny Smoothie

No recipe book could be without a little pumpkin pie number: Lots of ice has been added to this to thin it a little, so it's a really great thirst-quenching smoothie. With some added omega 3 and protein from the flax seeds, this would be a great post workout, holiday drink. Make sure you are using pure pumpkin for this and not a pumpkin pie mix that can be full of sugar!

Ingredients
- ¼ cup of pumpkin puree (from a can is fine)
- 2 cups of ice cubes
- ½ tsp maple syrup
- ½ cup of almond milk (unsweetened)
- ¼ tsp mixed spice
- ¼ tsp ground cinnamon
- 1 tsp flax seed

Instructions
1. Add all the ingredients to a blender and blend until smooth.

2. Sprinkle with a little more dusting of cinnamon if you like.

Raspberry Cream Protein Smoothie

Who doesn't like raspberries? This is so refreshing and light, with some great protein from some added chia seeds. It looks really pretty too.

Ingredients
- 1 cup frozen raspberries (reserve a few for decoration)
- 1 cup coconut yoghurt (no added sugar)
- 1 cup coconut milk (no added sugar)
- 1 tsp chia seeds

Instructions
1. Add all of the ingredients to a blender and blend until smooth.

2. If you are someone who really dislikes raspberry seeds, leave the chia seeds out when blending and pass the mix through a sieve. Add the chia seeds to the mix and wait for them to thicken and soften for 10 minutes.

3. Serve with some frozen raspberries bobbing about.

Brussel Muscle

Brussel Sprouts are surprisingly high in protein for a little green vegetable. They are part of the same family as kale, cabbage, broccoli and cauliflower and contain many health benefits. Using them in a smoothie is a great way to ensure you get the best from them. There is a tendency to over cook them where most of the nutritional benefits are lost. Great for blood health, they provide a good boost of Vitamin K.

Ingredients
- 1 cup of brussel sprouts
- 1 handful of spinach
- 1 cup of almond milk or coconut milk
- 1 green apple

Instructions
1. Remove any really tough stalks from the brussel sprouts.

2. Add all of the ingredients to a blender and blend well until smooth.

Power Punch

If you are looking for a smoothie to replace a meal, or to have a snack, it really ought to provide you with all the great benefits a good meal would give you. Plenty of vegetables, a good source of protein, good fat and a little carbohydrate for some needed energy. This is the WILDEST of colors!

Ingredients
- 4 cubes of frozen spinach
- ½ small roasted pumpkin
- ½ avocado
- 1 cup coconut water
- 1 tbsp flax seeds
- 1 tbsp walnuts
- 2 nori sheets roasted and then crushed

Instructions
1. Place all of the ingredients in to the blender and prepare to be dazzled. This is a wonderful collection of proteins, fats, carbohydrate, vitamins and flavors, the best meal replacer!

My Kiwi Coffee

Strange one this...there's no coffee and there's no kiwi. However, you'll feel like you've had a coffee after you've drank it, it looks like a glass of kiwi and it will give you a good boost of vitamin C, like a kiwi would give you. What an enigma!

Ingredients
- 1 tsp matcha green tea powder
- ½ cup freshly squeezed orange juice
- 1 frozen banana
- 1 tbsp chia seeds
- 1 handful of ice cubes

Instructions
1. Place all of the ingredients, a part from the chia seeds in to a blender and blend until smooth.

2. Stir in the chia seeds before serving.

A Sugar Fix

Sometimes something naturally sweet is all you want. This is it: A glass of sweet, iciness that's a wonderful refresher on a summer's afternoon. As smoothies go, it's worth getting this recipe out to convince someone, especially a child, to give them a go. Who wouldn't like this?

Ingredients
- 1 cup frozen red grapes
- ½ cup frozen dark cherries
- 1 cup almond milk (unsweetened)
- ½ cup fresh strawberries
- a small handful of ice

Instructions
1. Put all the ingredients in to a blender and blend until smooth.

2. Serve with some extra ice and any frozen pieces of fruit.

Dark Chocolate "Milk Shake"

How could you refuse this? It looks unhealthier than it actually is, but don't tell anybody that!

Ingredients
- 1 banana (frozen if possible)
- 1 tsp raw cacao powder
- 1 cup almond milk (unsweetened)
- 1 tsp macadamia nut butter (use another if unavailable)
- ½ tsp maple syrup
- 1 tsp of coconut milk powder (optional, adds more creaminess though!)

Instructions
1. Whizz all the ingredients together in a blender.

2. Serve with a dusting of extra cocoa powder and an indulgent smile.

Nuttylicious

Nuts are full of so much goodness for the Paleo diet that having a smoothie packed with them is really going to set you up for the day.

Ingredients
- 1 banana, frozen if possible
- 1 tbsp of any nut butter
- 1 cup of any nut milk (plus extra if want to make thinner)
- 1 tsp sunflower seeds
- 1 tsp pumpkin seeds

Instructions
1. Place all the ingredients in to a blender and blend well, until smooth.

2. Add some extra milk if desired.

Tutti Fruitie

Full of fruit and loads of Vitamins A and C, a source of Vitamin B6, copper, folate and potassium. This smoothie will keep your immune function and energy levels topped up well.

Ingredients
- 1 cup diced mango
- 1 cup diced pineapple
- 1 cup hemp milk (or other seed or nut milk)
- ½ cup chopped strawberries

Instructions
1. Blend all of the ingredients together until smooth.
2. Serve with some extra chopped strawberries if liked.

Sweet Passion

Watermelon and passion fruit are such a lovely combination of sweetness with hints of a tropical climate. A sunny smoothie for a rainy Paleo day maybe?

Ingredients
- 1 cup watermelon sliced
- 2 passion fruits
- 1 cup pineapple or apple juice
- ½ cup coconut milk

Instructions
1. Place the watermelon in to a blender.

2. Halve the passion fruits and scoop the seeds in to the blender.

3. Add the juice and milk and blend.

4. Serve ice cold with ice cubes.

Sesame, Banana and Coconut Slush

Sesame seeds are a great source of Vitamin E. Packed with protein, iron and omega 3, they are known to remove toxins, balance hormones and help with healthy skin and hair. This smoothie is a really comforting flavor that is both refreshing and filling so a great meal replacer.

Ingredients
- 1 tbsp sesame seeds
- 1 tsp tahini
- 1 banana frozen
- ½ cup coconut cream
- Large handful of ice

Instructions
1. Place all of the ingredients in a blender.

2. Blend well until all of the ingredients are well mixed and smooth.

3. Add some more ice to serve if liked.

Vegetable Pie

If you love your vegetables, you will love this. With a creamy avocado base, the flavours are added to with some glorious fresh herbs that bring these vegetables to life! The taste of the Mediterranean in a smoothie!

Ingredients
- ½ avocado
- 1 cup filtered water
- ½ cup mixed herbs, oregano, mint and parsley
- ½ lemon juice
- a handful of mushrooms
- 1 tbsp cashew nut butter
- 3 green olives
- 2 frozen cubes of spinach

Instructions
1. Put all the ingredients in to a blender and blend until smooth.

2. Stir through some extra chopped herbs if you like, to give a lovely speckled effect.

Fish Cake Smoothie

Not for the faint hearted. This fishy smoothie is rammed with omega 3 and protein and a great meal replacement. Give it a go; you may just be surprised.

Ingredients
- 2 Nori Sheets roasted and crushed
- 1 cup coconut water
- ½ avocado
- 3 inch piece of zucchini
- handful of kale (thick stalks removed)
- 1 tsp flax seeds
- 1 tsp chia seeds
- 1 tbsp almond butter
- 1 tbsp ground almonds

Instructions
1. Put all the ingredients in to a blender and blend until smooth.

2. Serve with some of the roasted nori, torn in to crisps on the side.

Good Weed

Hemp is delicious: Nutty, grassy and sweet all in one mouthful. It's full of great nutrition too and certainly worth slipping in to a Paleo diet. Full of omega 3 and 6, antioxidants, Vitamins B1, B2, B6, Vitamin C, Vitamin D, calcium, fiber, iron and zinc, you may find this smoothie to be the most nutrient dense yet!

Ingredients
- 1 cup of hemp milk
- 1 tbsp hemp seeds (hulled)
- 1 tbsp almond butter
- 1 large handful kale (stalks removed)
- ½ cup small florets of broccoli
- ½ avocado

Instructions
1. Whizz these ingredients up in a blender until smooth.

2. Sprinkle some extra hulled hemp seeds on top if liked, for a little crunch.

Toffee Apple Smoothie

There is something so comforting about the flavor of toffee. Paleo diets can still enjoy this lovely caramel flavor from the dates and maca powder (a fantastic Peruvian root full of health benefits for women's hormones!).

Ingredients
- 1 apple
- 1 cup almond milk (unsweetened)
- ½ cup chopped dates (soaked in 2 extra tbsps of nut milk)
- 1 tsp maca powder
- 1 cup of chopped melon (not watermelon, any other kind)

Instructions
- Place all of the ingredients in to a blender and blend until smooth.

- Reserve a few thin slices of apple (rubbed with lemon) and serve as decoration.

Late Summer Smoothie

These flavors evoke memories of late summer walks, with a hint of autumn coming from the wind. Walnuts and cinnamon are such a perfect match, with a wonderful sweetness from the other ingredients.

Ingredients
- 1 small frozen banana
- 1 apple
- 1 cup blackberries
- ½ tsp maple syrup
- 1 cup of almond milk (unsweetened)
- ½ tsp cinnamon
- 1 tsp walnuts

Instructions
1. Place all of the ingredients in to a blender and blend until smooth.

2. Sprinkle on some extra cinnamon to serve it you like.

Rhubarb and Custard

This custard flavor is produced from the vanilla extract in this recipe. Make sure you use a good quality one that is not just "essence" as you won't get the depth of flavor and sweetness. Rhubarb is certainly an underused vegetable and a fantastic antioxidant.

Ingredients
- 1 cup almond milk, unsweetened
- 1 tsp vanilla extract
- 1 tsp maple syrup
- 13oz can of rhubarb (not in syrup), or poach your own.
- 1 cup of ice
- 1 tbsp cashew nut butter

Instructions
1. Add all of the ingredients in to a blender and blend until smooth.

2. Serve in an ice cold glass.

Key Lime Skinny Smoothie

A creamy lime smoothie with some great toasty flavor from the sesame seeds: maybe resembling the pastry of this traditional dessert?

Ingredients
- 1 lime Juice and Zest
- 1 cup of coconut yoghurt
- 1 frozen banana
- ½ tsp maple syrup
- 1 tbsp of the coconut cream from a can
- ½ tsp vanilla extract
- Toasted sesame seeds

Instructions
1. Add the lime zest and juice, coconut yoghurt, banana and maple syrup to a blender and blend until smooth.

2. Whisk the tbsp of coconut cream until it is thick and then dollop on the smoothie.

3. Sprinkle over the toasted sesame seeds.

Power To The Protein

Whoa, this one's a heavy going, meal in one! This smoothie is high in fiber and protein, with lots of calcium for healthy bones. The black beans and cacao powder give a great "chocolate" color to this great smoothie.

Ingredients
- ½ banana – frozen
- 1 cup almond milk
- 1 tsp cacao powder
- 2 dates
- 1 tsp tahini
- ½ tsp ground nutmeg
- ½ can of black beans – about 200g
- ½ tsp cocoa nibs to sprinkle on top, optional

Instructions
1. Place all of the ingredients to in to a blender and whizz until smooth and creamy.

2. Pour in to a glass and sprinkle with the cocoa nibs if using.

Power To The Vanilla Protein!

Another version of the protein packed meal replacement. This time it's using a combination of butter beans and vanilla extract, to create a "white chocolate" smoothie.

Ingredients
- ½ banana – frozen
- 1 cup almond milk unsweetened
- 1 tsp tahini
- 2 dates
- 1 tsp vanilla extract
- ½ tsp cinnamon
- ½ can of butter beans (or cannellini beans) approx. 200g
- ½ tsp maple syrup to drizzle on top, optional

Instructions
1. Place all of the ingredients in to a blender and whizz until smooth and creamy.

2. Pour in to a glass and drizzle with a little maple syrup if using.

The Purple Beast

This is Paleo antioxidant special. This is full of fruits known to assist the body to clear up some of those free radical cells running riot. It's a great cleansing smoothie that tastes great too.

Ingredients
- ½ cup blueberries
- ½ cup black plums
- ½ cup red grapes
- ½ cup blackberries
- 1 cup of coconut water
- ½ frozen banana
- 1 tsp chia seeds

Instructions
1. Place all of the ingredients in to a blend and blend until smooth.

2. Frozen halved grapes would be a great decoration to be bobbing around in the smoothie, plus they keep the drink super cold.

Ruby Red

This is such a pretty smoothie to be sipping on. Add some cocktail umbrellas and some extra ice and you'll have the perfect drink to be sharing!

Ingredients
- 1 cup strawberries
- 1/2 cup cranberries
- 1 cup coconut milk
- 1 tsp flax seeds
- handful of ice
- ½ tsp stevia

Instructions
1. Place all the ingredients in to a blender and bend until smooth.

2. Don't add the stevia if your cranberries are quite sweet already.

A French Summer

This one is a bit different than the usual smoothies we see. It's always good to mix the flavors up a bit, and this one does! Try it, just to ease the curiosity. The walnuts add some wonderful health benefits with its omega 3, manganese and copper.

Ingredients
- 2 ripe figs
- handful of walnuts
- 1 cup apple juice
- ½ cup coconut yoghurt
- 1 banana, frozen
- ½ tsp cinnamon
- ½ tsp stevia

Instructions
1. Place all the ingredients in to a blender and blend until smooth.

2. You might not need the stevia if your figs are oozing sweetness.

The Market Mix

This is when the market has become a little confused. Some sweet fruits, fresh green vegetables and some nutritious hemp all in the same smoothie, creating a protein filled, vitamin packed, nourishing smoothie.

Ingredients
- 1 Pear
- ½ Avocado
- ½ cup Broccoli florets
- 1.5 inch barrel of Cucumber
- 2 tsp hulled hemp seeds
- 1 small handful of fresh mint leave
- 1 cup coconut water

Instructions
1. Blend all of the ingredients until smooth.

2. Serve with some extra chopped mint on top.

Savory Notes

Nutritional Yeast is becoming more and more popular, and if you have a tub of it in your cupboard, you may understand why. A deep savory flavor, which adds something a little "different" to a smoothie for sure!

Ingredients
- ½ cup cauliflower florets
- 1 cup coconut water
- ½ cup broccoli florets
- 1.5 inch barrel of cucumber
- 1 tsp nutritional yeast
- ½ tsp garlic paste

Instructions
1. Place all of the ingredients in to a blender and blend until smooth.

2. Decorate with slithers of cucumber and ice.

Skin Cream

The avocado in this smoothie lends some super skin health with its Vitamin E, Omega 3 and fatty acids. Dates have been added for a natural sweetness that gives this smoothie a bit of a caramel hint.

Ingredients
- ½ medium avocado
- 2 inch barrel of cucumber
- handful of baby spinach
- 2 tbsps cashew nuts
- 4 fresh dates
- 1 cup coconut water

Instructions
1. Scoop the flesh out of the avocado and roughly chop.

2. Chop the cucumber in to smaller pieces.

3. Add the avocado, cucumber and all of the other ingredients in to a blender and blend until smooth.

Veggie Patch

Not a big eater of vegetables? This smoothie may be one for you then as it is a shot of all the great kale benefits with vitamin A, B-6, C, calcium, iron and magnesium. Whizz this up and serve in shot glasses. The added carrot adds a good sweetness to balance the greenery.

Ingredients
- ½ banana
- handful of kale (stalk removed)
- 1 medium carrot
- 2 inch barrel of cucumber

Instructions
1. Place all of the ingredients in to a blender and blend until smooth.
2. Serve in shot glasses.

Chest Health

This recipe uses a cup of licorice tea, which is known to have a soothing effect on chesty coughs and mucus from a cold. The avocado is the base here for this creamy smoothie and the chia seeds add some protein to help the body recover and repair.

Ingredients
- 1 cup of baby spinach leaves
- 1 cup of cold licorice tea
- ½ avocado
- ½ frozen banana
- 1 tsp chia seeds

Instructions
1. Add all of the ingredients in to a blender

2. Blend until smooth. This smoothie should be consumed immediately for the best benefits.

Caca Maca

This smoothie is great for women's hormones. The maca is a great addition to assist with mood swings and the cacao and tahini are rich in magnesium, which helps with muscle cramps.

Ingredients
- ½ banana, frozen
- 1 tsp maca powder
- ½ tsp cacao powder
- 1 tsp tahini
- 1 cup almond milk
- 1 tsp flax seeds

Instructions
1. Add all of the ingredients in to a blender and blend until everything is smooth.

2. Serve in an ice cold glass and sprinkle with a little more cacao powder if liked.

Anti-Inflammation

With ingredients all high in anti-inflammatory properties, this smoothie will be a great addition to a diet for those suffering from rheumatoid arthritis, hay fever, aching and swollen joints and other inflammatory conditions.

Ingredients
- 1/2 small banana
- 1 cup of mango pieces
- 1 cup almond milk unsweetened
- 1 tsp flaxseed
- 2 tsp fresh turmeric root or 1 tsp ground turmeric
- ½ tsp cinnamon

Instructions
1. Put all of the ingredients in to a blender and blend until smooth.

2. If you are using turmeric root, chop a little beforehand to make the blending easier.

The Green Coco Bomb

The anti-oxidant abilities of raw cacao powder, is really enhanced in this smoothie recipe by the addition of some wonderful green vegetables. The hemp and avocado add a good boost of good fats, important for joints and good cholesterol levels. This bomb is packed full of nutrition!

Ingredients
- Small handful of baby kale
- Small handful of baby spinach or beetroot leaves
- 1 tsp hemp seeds or hemp oil
- ½ avocado
- 1 tsp raw cacao powder
- ½ tsp vanilla extract
- 1 cup of coconut water

Instructions
1. Wash the kale and spinach, removing any really tough stalks from the kale.
2. Add all of the ingredients in a blender and blend until really smooth.
3. Serve immediately.

The Speckled Egg

Named after the spattering of omega-3 rich seeds throughout this yolk yellow smoothie and the protein you may have got from an egg, (if there was one in it), from the chia and flax seeds. This is a great addition to a diet where protein could be a little better.

Ingredients
- ½ banana
- 1 cup almond milk
- 2 tsp pumpkin seeds
- 1 tsp chia seeds
- 1 tsp flax seeds
- ½ tsp turmeric

Instructions
1. Add the seeds to a blender and start whizzing to break them down a little.

2. Add the banana, milk and turmeric and whizz until you see a speckled yellow smoothie appear!

Peach On a Beach

Imagine relaxing on a beach somewhere, soothed and comforted by the sounds of waves on the shore beside you. The ginger in this smoothie will provide you with a lovely sense of well being, whilst the sweet peach will give you a sense of holidays and happiness.

Ingredients
- 1 large peach
- 2 tsp tahini
- 1 cup of filtered water
- ½ carrot
- 0.5 inch piece of root ginger

Instructions
1. Halve the peach and remove the stone.
2. Roughly peel the carrot and ginger and chop.
3. Add all the ingredients in to a blender and blend until smooth.

The Energy Blend

Chia seeds are great boost to the energy levels and provide both protein and omega 3 to your diet. This smoothie would make a great post workout drink, especially after a long run where the body needs to restore glycogen stores. Pineapple has a very soothing effect on the stomach, so if you have really pushed yourself and feel a little nauseous, this is the drink for you.

Ingredients
- 1 tbsp chia seeds
- ½ small pineapple
- 1 cup of cranberries, fresh
- 1 cup of ice cubes

Instructions
1. Peel and cube the pineapple.
2. Add the rest of the ingredients in to the blender, including the ice.
3. Blend until smooth and drink immediately.

Sweet Earth

Beetroot is known for its sweetness, having one of the highest levels of sugar in a vegetable, and if you're on a paleo eating plan, this isn't one to use frequently. However, there are a great many benefits to beetroot with its folate, vitamin C and potassium, so may be a little bit of a good thing, from time to time, will go a long way.

Ingredients
- 1 beetroot
- 1 handful of beetroot leaves
- 1 handful of rocket leaves
- 1 cup of water – filtered if liked
- 1 celery stalk

Instructions
- Add all of the ingredients in to a blender.

- Blend until smooth and enjoy immediately for the best benefits from the ingredients.

Dragon Fire

Dragon fruit must be one of the most attractive of all the tropical fruits. With it's its deep pink skin and white speckled flesh, it's a feast on the eye. However, it's also a feast for the body with its immune boosting Vitamin C, great fiber content and its lycopene that is associated with cancer fighting abilities.

Ingredients
- 1 dragon fruit
- 1 lime
- 1 inch piece of ginger root
- ½ mild chili

Instructions
1. Peel the dragon fruit and roughly chop in to pieces.

2. Juice the lime

3. Roughly peel the ginger root and chop in to small pieces.

4. Remove the chili seeds from the chili and cut in to small pieces.

5. Add all of the ingredients in to a blender and blend until smooth.

Dragon Milk

Here's another smoothie with this lovely, dragon fruit ingredient. This time a selection of seeds has been added to pack some further nutrition in to this smoothie. Chia seeds and flax seeds are full of Omega 3 good fats and protein to really add some proper sustenance to this drink.

Ingredients
- 1 dragon fruit
- ½ banana
- ½ cup coconut milk
- 2 cup water, filtered if like
- 1 tsp chia seeds
- 1 tsp flaxseeds
- 1 tsp vanilla extract

Instructions
1. Peel the dragon fruit and roughly chop.

2. Add all of the other ingredients in to a blender and blend until smooth.

3. Drink immediately.

Juices

Sometimes we have a real thirst that a smoothie just can't manage for us. A thinner, more refreshing drink, full of thirst fuel and hydro nourishment, with vitamins and minerals can be another choice to add to the drink repertoire.

So, what are juices? These are drinks made from the juice of a fruit or vegetable and have been put through a process where the fiber has been removed. There are different sorts of juicers but they have the same thing in common, they keep all the beneficial vitamins and minerals intact, but remove the insoluble fiber.

Types of Juicers

Centrifugal Juicer – this is the most common design of juicer. A fast spinning blade spins against a mesh filter that separates the juice and pulp. This tends to be a cheaper option than other designs but it does have the disadvantage that the heat generated from the fast moving blade does break down some of the nutritional benefits from the juice. It also doesn't provide such a good yield of juice.

Cold Press Juicer/Slow Juicer – This design is a newer concept, where the juice is extracted first by pressing and then crushing the fruit or vegetable. It gets more juice from the ingredients, so a better yield. It also doesn't create any heat, so the nutrients of the ingredients used are kept to their maximum. This design tends to be more expensive.

There are a number of new designs always appearing on the market, so research and find what suits you and your kitchen the best. Horizontal Single Auger, Vertical Auger, Twin Gear or Triurating and a champion juicer! You could go juicer crazy if you like?

You could just go back to basics and use an old fashioned method of blending the ingredients and soaking the contents through a cheesecloth over a bowl? It may be a good way to see how much you love the Paleo friendly Juice recipes coming up, before investing.

The benefits of juices are –
- They can provide you with your 5-a-day target easily.
- They will fill your body with an amazing array of micronutrients.
- They can be excellent in a weight loss plan as they still give you the vitamins and minerals but in less calories.
- Increases your energy as your body has an abundance of nutrients ready to be used from the juices.
- Your immune function will be greatly improved with the increase in vitamins from fresh sources
- They are a great way to fill your body with antioxidants, to help aid body functions providing detoxification.

The not so good benefits include –
- Juices can produce rapid spikes in blood sugar levels due to the fruit or vegetable being consumed without the fiber.
- Even though they make up less calories and can assist in weight loss, they don't fill you up as long and hunger will return.

- Juicers can be expensive.
- Juicers can be difficult to clean.

There is a place in your life for both juices and smoothies. Try some of these great flavor juice combinations and start filling your body with some extra nutrition!

All juices make 1-2 servings (unless specified). Ensure all of your ingredients are as cold as possible for the best results.

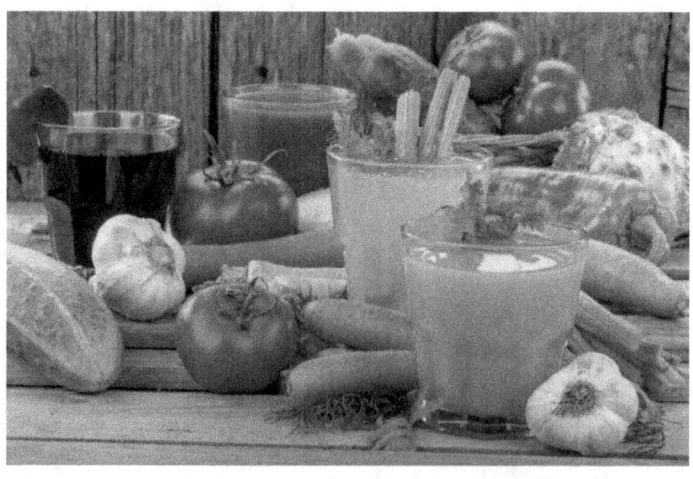

Refresher

A cucumber is a great addition to a juice, it's quite versatile, offering both sweet and savory notes and adds a huge dose of hydration with it's high water make up.

Ingredients
- 1 medium pear
- ½ cup of broccoli florets
- 2 inch barrel of cucumber

Instructions
1. Juice the pear, broccoli floret and cucumber.

2. Serve in an ice cold glass with slithers of cucumber.

Natures Pack Up

This juice is an example of how lucky we are to have such a sweet collection of fruits available to us! Do we really need all of that refined sugar addition? Watercress and asparagus has been added to add a balance of peppery earthiness that acts as a great companion to all of that natural sweetness. Honest!

Ingredients
- 1 green apple
- 8 green grapes
- ¼ honeydew melon (or galia)
- small handful of watercress
- 6 sprigs of asparagus

Instructions
1. Snap the woody stems off the asparagus and add to the juicer with the watercress.

2. Juice the remaining ingredients and combine well.

Sweet Earth

Root vegetables can really add a sweet flavor to a juice. A good fill of greenery with the peppery arugula adds some wonderful Vitamin K and calcium to this drink.

Ingredients
- 2 small carrots
- 2 parsnips
- 2 celery sticks, with leaves
- 1 handful of arugula

Instructions
1. Juice the ingredients.

2. Serve in an ice cold glass with extra ice cubes.

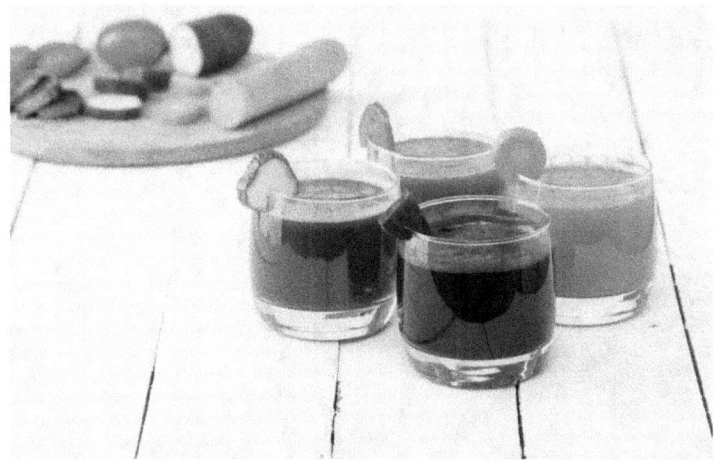

Cool As

Where did the phrase "cool as a cucumber" come from? Maybe the fact a cucumber can remain approximately 11.1 degrees cooler than the outside temperature it sits in. Probably due to it's high water content! How about grabbing some of that cool hydration and enjoying this great juice?

Ingredients
- 3 sticks of celery
- 2.5 inch barrel of cucumber
- 1 small fennel bulb
- 1 garlic clove
- handful of parsley or mint

Instructions
1. Juice the ingredients together.

2. Serve with some extra fresh herbs, shredded and sprinkled on top.

Heat Me Up

Ginger and a hint of chili? Have you ever wondered how some of the countries with the hottest climates in the world can use such heat producing ingredients? Did you know that there is a theory that the heat from a chili is able to raise your inside temperature to meet the outside temperature, causing you to sweat; and it's this sweat that your body produces that cools you down. Not convinced? Maybe a cold shower is your preferred choice! Either way, this juice is a nutritionally great, stimulating drink to perk you up.

Ingredients
- 1 garlic clove
- ½ red pepper
- 2 large tomatoes
- 1 large carrot
- 1.5 inch piece of root ginger
- Pinch of chili powder

Instructions
1. Juice the ingredients (except the chili) and blend.

2. Stir in as much chili powder as you dare!

3. Top with some crushed ice.

Fruitful Fields

The parsnip and carrot are so easy to grow that it would be the perfect place to find your ingredients...in your own garden! The apple tree would provide that sweet green apple and unless you live in a rather hot climate, maybe the melon needs to come from a supermarket shelf. Growing your own produce really is a satisfying hobby and could create some fantastic hydration inspiration for a paleo diet.

Ingredients
- 1 small parsnip
- 2 carrots
- ¼ galia melon (or other sweet flesh one)
- 1 small green apple

Instructions
1. Juice the ingredients together.

2. Serve with ice cubes and apple slices, rubbed with lemon.

Great Scott

This juice will provide you with a great drink to amaze you! The kale and spirulina will blast you with energy boosting iron and protein and a plethora of vitamins that will keep your body working at it's best. This is hardcore juice!

Ingredients
- 2 small carrots
- handful of radishes (tops removed)
- 1 parsnip
- handful of kale
- 1 tsp spirulina

Instructions
1. Juice the ingredients together.

2. Serve in shot glasses and down in one.

Strawberry Refresher

Peppermint is a much milder herb to use than the usual mint. Try and find this, or even another original flavor that seem to be on the increase at garden centers. Pineapple mint, horsemint, ginger mint and apple mint are all rather interesting varieties popping up at the moment so have a look round.

Ingredients
- 1 cup of strawberries
- 1 medium bunch of peppermint leaves
- 1.5 inch barrel of cucumber

Instructions
1. Place all of the ingredients in to a juicer and juice.
2. Serve in a short glass with extra peppermint leaves.

Where's The Orange?

There's lots of beta-carotene in this wonderful juice that will give you a great boost of antioxidants. These ingredients will also be supplying you with an abundance of Vitamin A, so drink up!

Ingredients
- 1 orange bell pepper
- 2 carrots
- 3 apricots
- 1.5 inch piece of root ginger

Instructions
1. Push all the ingredients through the juicer.

2. Add some ice cubes to some pretty glasses and serve ice cold.

Raspberry and Mango Punch

Raspberries are great for regulating your metabolism and fighting a number of diseases. Combined with mango and some fresh mint, this juice will provide a great boost to the immune system too.

Ingredients
- 1 cup of raspberries
- ½ large mango
- 1 small sprig of fresh mint

Instructions
1. Wash the fruit and herbs and push through a juicer.

2. Serve with lots of ice and extra mint leaves.

Hot Apple Shot

Horseradish is an ingredient that has a long history of being linked to medicinal aid. It has both antibiotic and antibacterial properties and in particular, offers protection against food borne pathogens. Before the days of refrigeration, horse radish was traditionally served a long side fish and meats as an insurance policy against these pathogens! Take this in a neat shot to combat a number of harmful bacteria's.

Ingredients
- 2 green apples
- 0.5 inch disk of wasabi or horseradish
- 1 small handful of mint

Instructions
1. Put all of the ingredients in to a juicer.
2. Serve in small shot glasses and take it in one!

Italian Fashion

Sweet, Italian and Paleo friendly. No pasta in sight, just an array of summery vegetables. The pepper will certainly help towards a healthy immune system, so if you can source these ingredients through the colder months (maybe find some tin tomatoes if the tomatoes are looking a bit green and hard), make it a regular addition to your juice repertoire.

Ingredients
- 1 red bell pepper, deseeded
- 2 large tomatoes
- 1 cup of white cabbage
- 1 tbsp fresh chopped oregano.

Instructions
1. Juice the pepper, tomatoes and cabbage.

2. Mix in in the chopped oregano and serve with a wedge of lemon in a short glass.

Green Queen

When you see a vibrant, green juice, you can only assume it MUST be good for you. That's exactly what this is, healthy, green and surprisingly tasty. There are studies showing that broccoli contains both cancer fighting and immune boosting properties so a great vegetable to get in to the juicer.

Ingredients
- 1.5 inch barrel cucumber
- ½ cup of broccoli florets
- 1 celery stick
- 2 small zucchini
- ½ lime, juice only
- 1 tsp spirulina

Instructions
1. Juice all of the ingredients together.
2. Serve with a lime wedge and plenty of ice.

Vegging Out

More and more of us turn to less sweet ingredients to provide the micronutrients available from our 5 a day target. A juice full of only vegetables will have less impact on your blood sugar levels so making it a great choice for those who tend to get sugar dips during the day. The fennel seed addition creates a really refreshing flavor.

Ingredients
- 1/2 cup cauliflower
- 1 carrot
- 1 parsnip
- 1 tomato
- 1 zucchini
- Ground fennel seeds

Instructions
1. Juice the ingredients together.
2. Serve with fennel seeds sprinkled on top.

Sweet and Sour

Sweet and sour flavors bouncing off one another, creates a real adventure for your taste buds. The lemon and grapefruit could create some real face twitching moments without the added mellow, sweet tones of the potato and peach. The grapefruit is known for its heart protecting properties and antioxidant ability.

Ingredients
- 1 grapefruit
- 1 small sweet mandarin
- ½ lemon juice only
- 1 peach

Instructions
1. Peel the grapefruit and mandarin. Juice the ingredients together for a really refreshing juice.

2. Serve with a wedge of lemon and lots of ice.

Chill On A Sunday

We all have probably fallen into an over indulged Sunday lunch time and ended up lounging around, feeling rather uncomfortable for a while. Chamomile is known for its calming effect on the body, both for the stomach and the mind. So, sip on this juice, relax and get a good nights sleep, ready for another Monday.

Ingredients
- 1 cup chilled chamomile tea
- 1 fennel bulb
- 1 lemon
- 1 apple

Instructions
1. Peel the skin off the lemon
2. Juice the rest of the lemon with the fennel and apple.
3. Blend with the tea, or stir well in to the juice.
4. Serve with crushed ice in a tall glass.

Fun Sun

These sunny flavors are full of Vitamin C. This vitamin is a super antioxidant and a great immune boosting micronutrient. Also high in Vitamin K, this juice is a great aid for healthy blood and it's essential blood clotting job.

Ingredients
- 1 orange
- 1 mango
- ½ pineapple
- ½ lime, juice only

Instructions
1. Juice all of the ingredients and

2. Serve in an ice cold glass, plenty of ice, and a cocktail umbrella!

Currant Brigade

There are a number of variety of currants out there to investigate. Red, black and white are all hugely popular in drinks and garnishes. Quite tart in taste, you may need to add the stevia, or a bit more for your palate. The 10 grapes added for the balance of sweetness here may not be enough! Packed with Vitamin C, these late summer berries will get you prepared for the cooler weather.

Ingredients
- ½ cup red currants
- ½ cup black currant
- ½ orange juice only
- 10 black grapes
- ½ tsp stevia if needed

Instructions
- Juice the ingredients together.

- Stir in a sweetener if a little too sour for your taste!

"Corrr"dial Please

A long, refreshing glass of something is sometimes just what you need after some exertion in the warmer weather. This juice is diluted with water to create a lighter drink to down.

Ingredients
- 2 large oranges
- 1 cup raspberries
- 10 grapes
- 1 cup filtered water

Instructions
1. Juice the fruit.

2. Use the water to dilute the juice.

3. Serve with a large helping of crushed ice, in a tall glass and straws.

Kernel Colonel

A lovely deep, sweet flavor from these fruits all containing a kernel. These drupes are sources of magnesium, which are essential for our wellbeing. Encouraging proper muscle function, regulating blood sugar and crucial for your immune system, this juice will be providing you with both taste and health.

Ingredients
- 4 apricots
- 2 small plums
- 1 peach
- 1 cup of filtered water
- Mint sprig for garnish

Instructions
1. Juice the apricots, plums and peach together.

2. Dilute with the water and enjoy with sprigs of mint.

Citron Whizz

This juice is great cleanser with a good helping of Vitamin C. Both the lemon and lime contain Limonene, which is a great phytochemical that can help increase the levels of enzymes that detoxify carcinogens

Ingredients
- 1 lemon
- 1 lime
- 12 green grapes
- ½ tsp stevia

Instructions
1. Juice the lemon, lime and grapes together

2. Add the stevia to taste.

3. Serve with wedges of extra lime and lemon with ice in a tall glass.

Christmas Cheer

When our normal diet gets turned upside down at Christmas, it's good to have this recipe up your sleeve. Full of Christmas flavor with the cinnamon and cranberries, sweetened by a good helping of melon and then with even more immune boosting Vitamin C from the orange, feel comforted by the fact your body will still get a boost of goodness.

Ingredients
- 1 cup cranberries
- 1 orange
- 1 cup chopped cantaloupe melon
- ½ tsp cinnamon

Instructions
1. Juice the cranberries, orange and melon together.
2. Mix in the cinnamon.
3. Serve with a cinnamon stick for a bit of Christmas fun.

Boost To The Moon

Kiwis and oranges together will give you a huge helping of Vitamin C, that will fill you with energy and well being. Juicing these two is an excellent way to get this essential vitamin in to your body, if you aren't too keen on the peeling issues with them both (did you know the kiwi skin is edible though?).

Ingredients
- 2 kiwis
- 2 oranges
- 1 apple

Instructions
1. Juice the ingredients together.

2. Serve this shot of vitamin C in a short glass and extra orange or kiwi slices.

Summer Sweetheart

How can anyone resist the simple sweetness of a drink filled with a cup full of juicy strawberries? Strawberries are known to contain ellargic acid, which is associated with great health benefits that fight ageing, neurological disease, cancer and inflammation.

Ingredients
- 2 kiwis
- 1 cup strawberries
- ¼ galia melon

Instructions
1. Juice these ingredients.

2. Add plenty of extra ice to the glass

3. Serve to a first time "juicer" and they'll be running to the next shop for their own Juicer!

Serene Dream

With the chamomile and the alkaline supply from the kiwi, you are bound to get a good nights sleep after this juice. May be save this juice recipe for a day when stress has really given you a good pounding.

Ingredients
- 2 kiwis
- 1 orange
- 1 apple
- 1 cup of cold chamomile tea

Instructions
1. Juice the kiwis, orange and apple together.
2. Stir in the chamomile tea and plenty of ice.
3. Serve in glass mugs.

Traffic Lights

Aptly named after the number of colors rammed in to the juicer for this recipe. It is known that the wider variety of colors we eat, the more chances are that we will get all of the nutrients our bodies need to thrive. Using a juicer is the perfect way to manage this with ease.

Ingredients
- ½ grapefruit
- 1 orange
- 1 kiwis
- 1 apple
- small handful of raspberries
- ½ lemon juice only

Instructions
1. Juice the ingredients together for a great flavor combination.

2. Try your own variation with this, just add 5 fruits containing different colors have fun with the tastes it creates.

Turkish Delight

With an abundance of sun, Turkey can produce such sweet fruits. If you can't find a quince, just use a green apple. The quince has long history of being cultivated in Asia and around the Mediterranean and it belongs to the same family as the apple and pear. Adding an astringent taste, this is a new flavor to experience! But this would be just as tasty without.

Ingredients:
- 1 pomegranate
- 1/2 quince (if not available, use 1 green apple)
- 1 cup cherries (morello if possible)
- 1 cup water melon
- ½ lime juice only

Instructions
1. Scoop out the pomegranate seeds.

2. Juice the seeds with the other ingredients.

3. Serve in pretty colored glasses with crushed ice.

Plum Punch

It is possible that the plum may have been one of the first fruits to be domesticated by humans. Remains have been documented to have been found in Neolithic settlement sites, so an ancient little fruit! It is estimated that up to 40 species of plum exist, so find your favorite!

Ingredients
- 4 small red or black plums
- 1 kiwi
- 1 apricot
- 1 cup of filtered water

Instructions
1. Juice the fruit ingredients together.

2. Mix with the water for a tall drink. Best served as chilled as possible.

Eastern Love

This sweet juice, is full of prebiotics, which help feed the good bacteria in our gut. There are many studies to show that the more good bacteria we have, the healthier we are, so it will pay to feed what you have!

Ingredients
- 1 fig
- 10 black grapes
- 2 small plums

Instructions
1. Juice all of the ingredients together.

2. Pour in to a tall glass and serve ice cold.

Mellow Yellow

The lychee is packed full of health benefits and a lovely flavor to add to a juice. It contains an important compound called Oligonol, which is known to aid blood flow, can assist in reducing weight and can also help protect skin against the sun's harmful UV rays.

Ingredients
- ½ grapefruit
- 1 cup lychees
- ¼ small galia melon
- 1 apple

Instructions
1. Juice the ingredients together.
2. Serve with wedges of lemon to bring the yellow to life!

Heat Sauce

Not for the faint hearted this one. A fantastic sweetness from the pepper, tomatoes and carrot, a refreshing addition with the celery, but then the pungent kick of a Tabasco and garlic combination. Yum, a juice to wake you up!

Ingredients
- 1 pepper (seeds removed)
- 2 tomatoes
- 1 carrot
- 1 celery stick
- Tabasco Sauce
- Garlic paste

Instructions
1. Juice the pepper, tomatoes, carrot and celery.

2. Stir in a dash of Tabasco (go easy!).

3. Whisk in the garlic paste and feel the benefits of the wake up in a glass! (Maybe follow this one with a Mint Shot!)

Mint Shot

A quick shot to wake you up, fill you with "zing" and help with any garlic or chili breaths lingering…

Ingredients
- Large handful of mint leaves
- ½ lemon
- 2 inch barrel of cucumber
- ½ cup coconut water to mix

Instructions
1. Juice the leaves and cucumber together.

2. Mix with the coconut water and serve in a small shot glass.

A Good Start

A breakfast juice that has the intense sweetness of the prune can really be a great start to the day. The spinach and spirulina provide a great addition of vitamins, iron and protein and if you run out of time to make a breakfast, you may just be forgiven with this quick juice – bet you won't miss that coffee.

Ingredients
- ½ cup of prunes
- 1 tsp spirulina
- handful of spinach
- 1 apples
- 1 pear

Instructions
1. Juice the ingredients together.

2. Add this drink to your morning breakfast table with a quinoa based porridge, extra fruit and seeds.

Strawberry Stars

The star fruit is a great exotic fruit that oozes Vitamin C. It also provides an array of B Vitamins, which are essential for our metabolism and hormone function. It can be a little tart, so the sweetness of the strawberries and melon balance this well.

Ingredients
- 1 cup strawberries
- 1 star fruit
- ½ galia melon

Instructions
1. Juice the ingredients together.

2. Serve with a slice of extra star fruit.

Sweetest Leaf In The Drawer

The iceberg lettuce has the least nutrients out of all of the lettuce leaves, but it's definitely the sweetest. It also has the highest number of calming properties, so if you're feeling run down or stressed, this is a juice for you.

Ingredients
- 1 apple
- 1 orange
- 1 lemon
- 1 handful of iceberg lettuce

Instructions
1. Quarter the apple.
2. Peel the orange.
3. Peel the lemon.
4. Juice all of the ingredients together and enjoy in a tall glass.

Friendly Monster

Fermented foods are really being promoted in the food media. Their association with increased good gut bacteria, good health, thinner bodies and sound well being are seeing an increase in the production of foods like sauerkraut, kimchi and kefir. These are the products that aren't pasteurized though, so try not to buy the long shelf life sauerkraut for this recipe. Try and source the live, unpasteurized version if you can and get maximum benefit from this wonderful ingredient.

Ingredients
- 1 apple
- 1 lemon
- ½ cup mooli
- 1 tbsp sauerkraut

Instructions
1. Quarter the apple
2. Peel the lemon
3. Add all of the ingredients in to a juicer.
4. Serve cold immediately.

Friendly Monster Mini

Like the above recipe, this juice uses some great fermented ingredients. With this one, this juice is a rammed full of goodness "shot" to be downed in one. A great power punch of energy, fuel, protein and some probiotics to really look after you stomach.

Ingredients
- 1 handful of baby spinach
- 1 tbsp sauerkraut
- A small bunch of parsley leaves
- 1 apple
- 1 tsp spirulina

Instructions
1. Place all of the ingredients in to a juicer, apart from the spirulina.

2. Whisk in the spirulina.

3. Serve this juice in small shot glasses, gulping down in one to give you a great start to whatever day you have planned!

Hot Tomato

Tomatoes contain a good supply of lycopene, which is known for it's anti-cancer properties. Even though cooked tomatoes contain more of this cancer busting substance, this raw tomato juice will still deliver a great deal of benefits. It has been added to by a kick of chili and sweetness of some red bell pepper, which both contain capsaicin, known to have an ability to suppress tumor growth, so drink up and enjoy!

Ingredients
- 4 tomatoes
- ½ red chili
- ½ red pepper

Instructions
1. Make sure all of the seeds are removed from the pepper and chili.

2. Add all of the ingredients in to a juicer.

3. Serve ice cold.

Super Juice

Coriander is full of manganese, iron and magnesium and is one of those flavors you love or hate. Give this one a go with the pineapple and ginger as the taste really changes to something quite unique and it loses the "soapiness" that some associate with it.

Ingredients
- 1.5 inch piece of root ginger
- 1 1/2 cups of pineapple
- 1 small bunch of coriander

Instructions
1. Juice all of the ingredients together.

2. Serve with a handful of ice and an open mind!

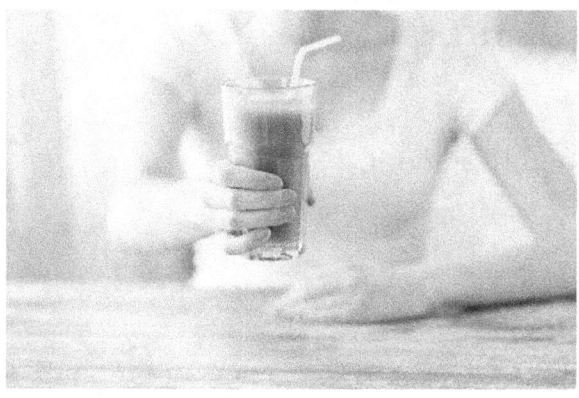

Tummy Treat

This recipe uses Hemp oil, which is great ingredient to add to a smoothie or juice. It contains both Omega 3 and Omega 6 oils were are essential for our well being. It has quite a nutty, grassy flavor, which some people adore. With the sweetness from the orange and carrot here, you may not taste it very much anyway, but you'll be getting all the benefits.

Ingredients
- 1 orange, juice only
- 1 small carrot
- 2 tomatoes
- 1 celery stick
- 1 tsp hempseed oil
- 1 cup of filtered water

Instructions
1. Juice the orange, carrot and tomatoes

2. Add these to a blender with the celery stick, water and hempseed oil.

3. Blend until smooth.

Parsley Pulse

Working with protein, the Vitamin K in parsley can really strengthen bones and improve blood health. This is quite a "herby juice" so try and pack the leaves between the heavier items to get as much juice from them as possible.

Ingredients
- 1 handful of parsley leaves
- 1 fresh rosemary sprig
- 1 garlic clove
- 6 green beans
- small handful of baby spinach leaves
- 2 inch barrel of cucumber
- 1 celery stick
- 1 tsp hemp oil and chilled water to add

Instructions
1. Juice all of the ingredients a part from the hemp oil and water.

2. Add the juice to the hemp oil and whisk.

3. Add ice cold water to taste and top up with ice cubes.

Stress Reducer

Celery, celery leaves, seeds and celeriac are known to reduce the stress hormone called cortisol in our bodies. This juice is a great de-stresser and is a good choice for an after work aperitif.

Ingredients
- 2 celery stalks, with leaves if possible
- 1 apple
- small matchbox size piece of celeriac
- ½ tsp hemp oil

Instructions
1. Juice all of the ingredients together

2. Add the hemp oil and give a good stir to the juice

3. Serve ice cold

Herbal Infusions: Teas and Tisanes

Just to clear up any confusion as to what's what here. These two elements are a little different from one another and it's worth just taking a moment to get to know what we're talking about, just in case a tea guru comes along and wants to put you straight!

Teas are made using leaves from the tea bush, also known as Camellia sinensis. This can be green tea, white tea, black tea or oolong tea. These are all classed as proper tea but they're just processed differently. They can be served hot or cold.

A traditional tisane (or ptisan) is the term given to any other drink that has been made from any herbal infusion that has not used a tea leaf. They can also be served hot or cold and can make a lovely refreshing summer drink. Tisane's are also associated with the medicinal beverages that have been made from herbs and spices for particular ailments, ones that have a long standing history as being helpful for certain health issues.

The term "herbal tea", or "herbal infusion" is so wildly used to describe any tea nowadays that we're going to be very relaxed about this and we're just going to refer to the recipes as teas and infusions, but you know what's what!

Whichever term is used, there are two ways in which these great drinks can be made; by a "steeping" method and by a "decoction" method. These are good terms to blow away that tea guru that may pop up!

"Steeping" is a method where you bring water to a boil and then pour over the leaves or flowers of delicate herbs and leave to soak or "steep" in the water for about 5-20 minutes (depending on your herbs you are using). This method is much better for delicate plants as simmering would be too harsh.

The "decoction" method is when you boil a plant ingredient in water, reducing the liquid to intensify the flavor. It's usually done with herbs and spices in the form of stems, roots and seeds, as the active part of these ingredients are harder to extract. When gently boiled for up to 45 minutes, these herbs release these benefits and taste in to the water, which "steeping" would not do easily.

On another note here – a herbal infusion is also a label that could be given to any other sort of herbal mix. This could be anything; oils, vinegars, pastes, rubs, butters, creams for cooking with, syrups to add flavor to and there's a wealth of herbs and spices to choose from to make them with. But that's a different story!

There are a number of pots, balls and strainers on the market to enhance and make the natural tea making process really easy.

The Good Old Fashioned Tea Pot – With so many pretty designs on the market, we are spoilt for choice. Pour in boiled water, your choice of herb and then (if it doesn't contain it's own strainer inside) pour over a strainer in to a cup.

Tea Ball – A re-usable mesh ball to add to a pretty teapot. The flavors develop inside the pot and release the ingredient tastes in to the water. Not so good for large items you want to add to a tea.

Stainless Steel French Press – This works a bit like a coffee pot, where you add the water and herbs to the water inside, leave to steep and then push down a plunge strainer to keep the ingredients from going in to the cup.

The Silicone Re-Usable Tea Bag – Great for tea on the go! Add your favorite herbs, put in you bag and ask for a cup of hot water when you're out. Steep like you would normally. It's the perfect way to keep the natural hydration going all day long.

The Old English Tea Strainer – Maybe you are after a more refined tea affair. This is just a strainer that is placed over your cup, filled with the herbs you would like to use. Pour over the water and leave to steep, removing the strainer before drinking.

Back to hydration, the following recipes are a mix of teas and tisanes, light, delicate and refreshing. Some of these drinks are made by using a "decoction" method and some the "steeping" method. Find flavors you enjoy, try ones you like the sound of or use the ones you feel may help a certain well being issue you may have. These recipes use dried and fresh herbs and spices that are all readily available from your garden or good store. They make a great alternative to coffee and will keep your hydration well topped up. With some fantastic ingredients, rammed with health benefits, you really will be drinking yourself to a healthier you.

All recipes are for 1 serving, unless specified.

Cinnamon Tea

This is a simple tea that claims can help with weight loss. Cinnamon is known for it's antioxidant properties, but it is known to regulate blood sugar levels reducing the sugar cravings that cause over eating. It is also associated with speeding up metabolism so a great aid to weight loss. To keep this tea Vegan, use maple syrup or stevia to sweeten.

Ingredients
- 1 cup boiling water
- 1 tsp Ceylon cinnamon (or organic if you can't find this)
- 1 tsp stevia/1 tsp maple syrup.

Instructions
1. Mix the maple syrup or stevia with the cinnamon.

2. Stir in to the boiled water and leave to infuse for 10-15 minutes.

Slippery Elm and Ginger Settler

Slippery Elm is a tree native to North America and there is a long history of the bark of this tree being used for its medicinal properties. In particular, it has a soothing ability to deal with stomach complaints, such as diarrhea, constipation and also inflammation of the respiratory tract. With the ability to reduce bloating, this is a great drink to incorporate in to your hydration if you do suffer with digestive issues.

Ingredients
- 1 tsp slippery elm bark powder (available in most wholefood shops)
- 1 lemon
- 1 cup of boiling water

Instructions
1. Leave the water to cool slightly.

2. Half the lemon and squeeze half of the juice in to the cooling water.

3. Slice the other half of the lemon in to think slices and add to the water.

4. Stir in the slippery elm bark powder and leave to thicken for 5-10 minutes or so.

5. Drink immediately

Fenugreek, Lime leaf and Turmeric Tisane

Fenugreek is a spice used in many different ways through out the world. Whether ground in to other spices, used as a treatment for diabetes, pickling or creating relishes, it has a great many benefits to our health. Known to increase libido in men and reduce inflammation inside the body, it is certainly one to try.

Ingredients
- 1 ½ cups of water
- 1 tbsp fenugreek seeds
- 4 lime leaves
- 1.5 inch piece of fresh turmeric root
- 1 lemon grass stalk
- 1 slice of lemon to serve

Instructions
1. Bring the water to a boil.

2. Bash the fenugreek seeds a little, crush the lime leaves and cut the turmeric root. Squash the lemon grass too and add all of the ingredients in to the boiled water.

3. Leave to simmer gently for 15-20 minutes to really give the flavors a chance to release.

4. Serve with a slice of lemon.

Lemon and Ginger Tonic

Deliciously delicate, aromatic and refreshing, these flavors are a great combination for a great taste. Both are known to energize so it would be great tisane to get going in the morning for a fresh wake up!

Ingredients
- 1 cup water
- 1 inch piece fresh ginger root
- 10 lemon verbena leaves
- 1 slither of lemon peel
- (1/2 tsp stevia or maple syrup, optional)

Instructions
1. Boil the water

2. Roughly chop the ginger root and add to a tea ball or other tea strainer

3. Wash and roughly tear the lemon verbena leaves.

4. Add the leaves and lemon peel to the ginger.

5. Add the boiling water and leave to steep for 5-10 minutes, depending how strong you like it.

6. This can be enjoyed hot or cold.

Nettle Tea

Not just a nuisance in the garden, nettles have a long standing history of being used to treat painful muscles, eczema, arthritis, gout and anemia. Today they are known to treat urinary tract infections and problems during the early stages of an enlarged prostate so a great cup of tea for men.

Ingredients
- A good handful of nettles, careful how you handle them.
- 1 cup of water

Instructions
1. Boil the water

2. Place the nettle leaves in the water and leave to steep for 10-15 minutes.

3. The flavor and benefits would have released in to the water and the "sting" removed.

Cup Med

This deeply savory tea is a celebration of Mediterranean flavors. Oregano is known for its assistance with detoxifying the body with a rich helping of manganese. It helps energize the body and speed up metabolism with the Vitamin B it contains and boosts the immune system.

Ingredients
- 10 leaves fresh oregano (or 2 tsp dried oregano)
- 10 reeds of chives
- 5 mint leaves (or 1 tsp dried mint)
- 3 stems of lemon thyme (or normal thyme)
- 1 cup of water
- (1/2 tsp stevia or maple syrup, optional)

Instructions
1. Bring the water to the boil.
2. Wash all the herbs
3. Rip the oregano, chives, mint and scrunch up the thyme.
4. Add to a tea strainer and pour over the boiled water.
5. Leave to steep for 5-10 minutes depending how strong you like it.
6. Enjoy hot

Artichoke Tea

Artichokes are amongst the top 10 highest anti-oxidant rich foods. With a long standing history of combating various stomach complaints, such as irregular bowels and stomach upset it is also thought the "clean the blood". Added to with the delicate fragrance of lemon verbena, this slightly sweet tea is a real soother.

Ingredients
- 2 tbsp dried or fresh artichoke leaves
- 8-10 leaves of lemon verbena
- 1 cup of water

Instructions
1. Bring the water to a boil.//
2. Add the dried artichoke leaves and lemon verbena leaves to a tea pot or ball.
3. Leave to steep for 5-10 minutes.

Cardamom and Vanilla Tea

Cardamom contains a volatile oil called cineol, which is great to clear up chesty coughs and bronchitis type symptoms. It also boosts the metabolism and helps the body burn more fat, so definitely worth trying if you are on a weight loss goal.

Ingredients
- 1 tsp cardamom pods
- 1 tsp vanilla extract or ½ vanilla pod
- 1 cup of almond milk, unsweetened
- Pinch of cinnamon

Instructions
1. Bring the milk to a boil and leave to one side.
2. Crush the cardamom pods and add to the milk.
3. Stir in the vanilla extract or if using the pod, cut the ½ vanilla pod in half and add to the milk.
4. Leave to infuse in the warm milk for 10-15 minutes.
5. Strain through a tea strainer and enjoy warm with the pinch of cinnamon sprinkled on the top.

Herbal Feast Tea

This tea is a feast of many flavors and many health benefits. Working as a digestive aid, it can relieve bloating and stomach cramps. It can also work as a relaxant, easing tension and nervous headaches. Leave this tea to steep for as long as you like, depending on how strong you like it

Ingredients
- 8 mint leaves
- 3-4 fennel fronds
- 3-4 dill fronds
- small handful of parsley
- 1 cup of water

Instructions
1. Boil the water pour in a tea pot.

2. Add the mint leaves, fennel, dill and parsley to the water and leave to steep for 5-20 minutes, depending on our preference. Strain in to a cup or mug.

3. Enjoy with a few extra herbs added when serving.

Rosemary Tea

This herbal infusion is a warming winter drink, but is equally good in the summer if you love the flavor of this drink. Rosemary is full of unique compounds and oils that provide a number of antibacterial, antifungal and anti-inflammatory properties.

Ingredients

- 1 good sprig of fresh rosemary (or 2 tsp dried rosemary)
- 1 cup of water

Instructions

1. Strip the leaves from the stem of the fresh rosemary and chop the leaves roughly.

2. Boil the water.

3. Put the leaves or dried herbs in to a tea strainer, ball or pan.

4. Pour over the water and leave to steep for 5-10 minutes.

5. Strain and drink hot.

Turmeric, Lemon and Ginger Blend

Turmeric is a great addition to your drink as it is so well known for it's anti-inflammatory properties. It has been used in a medicinal capacity for thousands of years and promotes protection against oxidant damage. This tea is a great store cupboard drink, as both the ginger and turmeric can be used in powder form. Feel free to use both of these in their fresh root form though and gently boil for 30 minutes to release all the good benefits from them.

Ingredients
- ½ tsp ginger ground
- ½ tsp turmeric ground
- 3 slices of lemon
- 1 cup of water

Instructions
1. Boil the water

2. Place the ginger and turmeric in a mug and stir together.

3. Pour over the boiled water and stir in to the ground spices.

4. Mix well until dissolved.

5. Add the lemon slices and leave for the flavors to develop for 10 minutes.

6. Enjoy hot

Sleepy Turmeric Latte

Although not really a "tea", we had to add this to the herbal tea section, as you have to try this before bed one night! No caffeine, it's just a blend of creamy sweet almond milk, a dash of ginger and good helping of turmeric. This is almost guaranteed to produce a warm, relaxed mind for a good night's sleep.

Ingredients
- 1 cup almond milk (unsweetened)
- 1 tsp turmeric ground
- ½ tsp ginger ground

Instructions
1. Boil the milk

2. Stir in the turmeric and ginger and mix until dissolved and the milk has turned a lovely golden color.

3. Enjoy warm, 30 minutes before heading to bed.

Tranquillity

This herbal tea is to promote peace and calm and has some lovely aromatic zing from the lemon grass. You could add a pinch of stevia if you want to sweeten it up a little, although the chamomile does have a little sweetness anyway.

Ingredients
- 1 cup of water
- 1 lemon grass stalk
- 2 tsp chamomile

Instructions
1. Boil the water

2. Bash the lemon grass with a rolling pin or mallet to start releasing some of the flavor.

3. Put the lemongrass (cut if need be) in to a pot or tea ball with the chamomile.

4. Pour over the boiling water and leave to steep for 5-10 minutes. Add a pinch of stevia if you like.

Blackcurrant Leaf and Peppermint Tea

If you grown blackcurrants in your garden or know somebody that does, don't just use the currants! The leaves bring a lovely blackcurrant flavor when steeped and you could add some berries to the mix when serving if you like. The peppermint is a great lifting taste to add to the blackcurrant.

Ingredients
- 1 cup of water
- 8-10 blackcurrant leaves
- 8-10 leaves peppermint (or use a peppermint tea bag)
- Blackcurrants to serve, optional.

Instructions
1. Boil the water

2. Scrunch the blackcurrant leaves a little and add to a pot with the peppermint leaves or teabags

3. Pour over the boiling water and leave to steep for 5-10 minutes.

4. Serve with a few blackcurrant, oozing in the hot water.

Vanilla, Apricot and Mint Tea

Vanilla is always a favorite flavor for many people and it's full of some wonderful health benefits. Able to reduce inflammation and cholesterol, vanilla is perfect to enhance your wellbeing, bringing its comforting, sweetness. Its also known for its antioxidant abilities so good to assist your body with clearing up the free radical cells in our bodies.

Ingredients
- 1 cup of water
- ½ vanilla pod
- 1 apricot
- 8 leaves of mint leaves.

Instructions
1. Boil the water

2. Cut the vanilla pod, keeping the seeds inside*. Add to the pot or tea ball.

3. Wash, cut and remove the stone from the apricot. Cut in to quarters and add to the teapot or ball.

4. Pour over the boiled water and leave to steep for 5-10 minutes

5. Serve with fresh mint leaves.

*Tip

You could dry the vanilla pod out after drinking this tea and add to a jar of sugar. When kept like this, you can create some vanilla sugar to use for baking and get more out of this expensive ingredient.

Turmeric Orange Splash

This invigorating tea will provide your mouth with some good refreshment. Turmeric acts as a great anti-oxidant and the Vitamin C in the orange also adds to the boost in immune system. A great combination for a any time of the day drink.

Ingredients
- 2 cups water
- 1 inch piece of fresh root of turmeric
- 1 orange – just slithers of peel from the entire fruit
- 2 cloves

Instructions
1. Boil the water in a pan
2. Cut the turmeric up a bit and add to the pan.
3. Add the orange peel pieces and cloves to the pan.
4. Simmer for 20 minutes with a lid on.
5. Strain and enjoy hot or cold with ice.

Fennel Infusion

Fennel is a wonderful flavor and is known for its ability to relieve indigestion and soothe the stomach. This easy infusion is so simple to make and a great start to the day when you may feel a little delicate.

Ingredients
- 2 tsp fennel seeds
- 1 cup water

Instructions
1. Boil the water

2. In a pestle and mortar, bash the seeds to start releasing some of their flavor.

3. Add the boiling water and leave to steep for 15 minutes.

4. Strain and drink hot.

Sage and Onion "Broth"

Sage is traditionally known to uplift you! It can help deal with the PMS issues some women suffer with and also assist with symptoms from the menopause. This is really a savory tea that is an instant boost for you to enjoy.

Ingredients
1. 1 cup water
2. 8 sage leaves
3. 8 reeds of chives

Instructions
1. Boil the water
2. Wash and tear up the sage leaves
3. Wash the chives and chop in to 2 cm pieces
4. Add the herbs to a strainer or ball.
5. Pour over the water and leave to steep for 10 minutes
6. Enjoy hot

Hibiscus Blend

Hibiscus is a lovely floral, aromatic petal that produces some wonderful health benefits if you are suffering a bit with a sore throat or sore gums. It is also associated with reducing high blood pressure. And the color? Amazing!

Ingredients
- 1 tsp dried hibiscus leaves
- pinch of stevia (optional)
- pinch of dried rose petals
- 1 cup water

Instructions
1. Boil the water

2. Place the hibiscus, stevia (If using) and rose petals in to a tea pot and pour in the boiled water.

3. Leave to steep for 15 minutes.

4. Enjoy hot or cold.

Mint Twist

Mint is known for its ability to soothe an unsettled stomach. To add a twist on the flavor and to also further this ability to soothe, dill has been added to this drink. These flavors are a real change from the usual "peppermint tea" and make a great cup of settling benefits.

Ingredients
- 1 cup of water
- 2-3 fronds of fresh dill
- 8 leaves of fresh mint

Instructions
1. Boil the water
2. Wash the herbs
3. Rip the mint and roughly chop the dill.
4. Add to the herbs to a tea ball or pot.
5. Leave to steep for 5-10 minutes.
6. Enjoy warm

Raspberry and Mint Infusion

Raspberries are a great mix with mint. The color and flavor that steeps in to this drink will brighten you up and the soothing mint will start your day off well. Raspberries are full of great health benefits and have a high concentration of ellagic acid, a compound that could be useful in preventing the growth of cancer cells.

Ingredients
- 1 cup water
- handful of raspberries (can be frozen or fresh)
- 8 leaves fresh mint.

Instructions
1. Boil the water
2. Wash the mint and raspberries
3. Roughly tear the mint leaves and add to a cup or heat proof glass.
4. Add the raspberries.
5. Pour over the water and leave to steep for 15 minutes.
6. This can be enjoyed just warm or cold with lots of ice. Eat the raspberries as you drink for the best benefits!

Poppy Tonic

Poppy seeds have a known history to treat diarrhea. However, a tea made from the seeds is an age old remedy for anxiety and nervous tension. It's a great herbal tea to give someone during difficult time and can really help with worry.

Ingredients
- 1 tbsp poppy seeds
- 8 lemon verbena leaves
- 1 cup of water
- 1 slice of lemon to serve

Instructions
1. Boil the water

2. Place the poppy seeds and lemon verbena leaves in to the water and leave to steep for 10-15 minutes.

3. Serve with a slice of lemon.

Lemon and Tarragon Brew

Tarragon has a very strong flavor so test this drink before allowing it to steep for too long. With its anti-oxidant properties it can help to support cardiovascular health. Rich in magnesium, iron, zinc, calcium and Vitamins, A, C and B-6, this is a pretty sturdy addition to a cup of tea.

Ingredients
- 1 cup water
- 8 tarragon leaves
- 6 lemon verbena leaves

Instructions
1. Boil the water
2. Wash the herbs
3. Roughly tear the herbs and add to a cup or tea ball.
4. Leave to steep for 5-6 minutes.
5. Enjoy hot.

Spice Blend

Cumin seeds and coriander seeds are a comforting flavor and bring some strong health benefits to our wellbeing. Cumin has been associated with supporting the digestive system, lowering cholesterol, boosting immunity and acting as a great anti-oxidant, helping to mop up those free radical cells in our bodies.

Ingredients
- 2 tsp cumin seeds
- 2 tsp coriander seeds
- 1 cup of water

Instructions
1. Boil the water.

2. In a pestle and mortar, bash both the seeds up quite well to start releasing their flavor and aroma.

3. Add the seeds to a pot with strainer.

4. Add the water to the pot and steep for 15 minutes.

5. Drink hot.

Juniper Berry Tea

Juniper berries have some great properties to reduce indigestion and bloating after eating, so this tea may be a good after dinner drink. Also acting as a mild diuretic, it can stimulate urination too.

Ingredients
- 2 cups of water
- 2 tsp juniper berries
- 1 slither of lemon peel
- ½ tsp stevia

Instructions
1. Bring the water to a boil and bring to a gentle simmer.

2. Add the berries and lemon.

3. Cover and cook for 15 minutes.

4. Strain in to a mug.

5. Add the stevia to taste.

Ginseng Ginger Tea

Ginseng has a history of being used to treat fatigue – something we can relate to! Ginseng can promote good memory and attention spans and can be a great support for stress and anxiety. Ginger has been added to this drink, but you can still get the unique taste and sweetness from the ginseng.

Ingredients
- 2 tsp ground ginseng or 2 small roots
- 1 inch piece of fresh ginger root
- 2 cups of water
- 1 lemon slice
- Stevia to taste

Instructions
1. Bring the water to a boil in a pan.

2. Chop the ginger in to small chunks.

3. Add the ginseng and ginger to the pan and simmer, covered for 10 minutes.

4. Strain and pour in to mug.

5. Check for sweetness and add some stevia if needed.

6. Add the slice of lemon and enjoy hot.

Vanilla, Orange and Sage Remedy

Sage is a wonderful help for a sore throat. This tea will add some comfort to any soreness and some vitamin C to help the immune system fight back. The vanilla is a known anti-bacterial agent and will offer some support to get your back fighting fit. Remember, hydration is even more important when you're under the weather and drinking a tea with no caffeine will only add to your hydration.

Ingredients
- 1 cup of water
- ½ vanilla pod
- 8 sage leaves
- 1 small orange

Instructions
1. Boil the water.

2. Cut the vanilla, leaving the seeds intact. Add to a pot or tea ball.

3. Add the sage to the ball or pot.

4. Half the orange and slice in to pieces. Place in the pot or tea ball.

5. Pour on the water.

6. Squeeze the juice from the other half of the orange in to the pot.

7. Steep for 15 minutes and enjoy warm for the best throat comfort.

Elderberry and Cinnamon Tisane

Elderberry has a long standing history of being useful for coughs and colds; elderberries also support Eye and vision health. This plant imparts the smell of summer in to a mug and this drink is a delicately, floral brew to enjoy.

Ingredients
- 1 cup of water
- 1 handful of elderflower blossom
- ½ tsp Ceylon cinnamon
- Stevia to taste

Instructions
1. Boil the water

2. Add the elderflower blossoms to a pot or tea ball.

3. Add the water

4. Stir in the cinnamon.

5. Leave to steep for 5-10 minutes until the flavors have developed.

6. Strain and adjust sweetness if need be with the stevia.

Lavender Soother

Lavender is quite a strong, floral flavor so don't put too much in. It's known for its calming properties, promoting relaxation and sleep so it would be shame to not include this in a tea recipe for our well being.

Ingredients
- 8 leaves of lemon verbena
- 1 tsp lavender flowers (dried or fresh)
- 1 cup of water
- Slice of lemon to serve, optional

Instructions
1. Boil the water

2. Add the lemon verbena and lavender flowers to a pot or tea ball.

3. Add the water

4. Leave to steep for 5-10 minutes

5. Enjoy warm with a slice of fresh lemon if liked.

Celery Seeds and Basil Cup

Celery seeds are not known so readily but have the most gloriously bold, salty flavor. This "tea" could almost be a broth! The basil adds a lovely fresh hit to the celery. Celery seeds are great for your health and a brilliant stand by in the kitchen cupboard. They have been used for many years to assist with poor digestion and today, as a diuretic.

Ingredients
- 1 cup of boiling water
- 8 basil leaves
- 1 tsp celery seeds
- 1 slice of lemon

Instructions
1. Heat the water to a boil.
2. Wash the basil leaves.
3. Tear the basil leaves up roughly and add to a pot.
4. Pour on the water and stir in the celery seeds.
5. Leave to steep for 10-15 minutes.
6. Serve hot with the lemon slice.

Parsley, Mint and Lemon Tisane

Parsley has a lot of benefits and is readily available in dried and fresh varieties. It's such a versatile herb that it's worth investing in a large pot of it and place in on the kitchen window. It can be added to cooking and of course, this drink. Parsley contains vitamin A, C and K and has evidence to suggest it can prevent kidney stones.

Ingredients
- 1 cup water
- 8 leaves of fresh parsley
- 8 leaves of mint
- 1 lemon – slithered peel only

Instructions
1. Boil the water
2. Wash the herbs and prepare the lemon.
3. Roughly tear the leaves and place in a tea strainer, pot, or ball.
4. Pour over the water
5. Leave to steep for 15 minutes.
6. Enjoy hot or cold

Green Tea and Tonic

Green tea is known for its health benefits. Created from the same tea leaf that creates the usual cup, it is grown in slightly different areas, harvested and processed in ways that keep the tea leaf close to its natural state . Containing $1/4^{th}$ of the caffeine that coffee has, this a good compromise to eliminate caffeine from your diet and could be good step towards becoming free of caffeine altogether. With some beneficial herbs added to this infusion, it's a great breakfast cup to give you a little lift first thing.

Ingredients
- 1 cup of water
- 1 green tea bag
- 10 fresh marjoram leaves

Instructions
1. Boil the water.

2. Place the marjoram leaves and green tea bag in the water and leave to gently infuse for 5-10 minutes.

3. Drink this uplifting tonic in replace of a cup of coffee first thing when you get up, as a first step to reducing your coffee.

A Noble Brew

This tea is full of a garden of herbs. Aromatic, fragrant and savory that will give your taste buds a real work out. If you have your own herb garden, pick as many of these as you have and add others if you like. Herbs have such wonderful flavors that can really help you unwind and feel some positive relaxation, dreaming of garden walks, flowers and warming days.

Ingredients
- 1 cup of water
- 1 sprig of thyme
- 4-5 needles of rosemary
- 4-5 leaves of fresh mint
- 4-5 leaves of oregano
- 3-4 flowers from a lavender bush
- 2-3 chive flowers

Instructions
1. Bring the water to a boil.//
2. Wash all of the herbs.
3. Place in to a tea pot and pour over the boiled water.
4. Leave to infuse for 5-10 minutes.
5. Pour through a strainer and enjoy a taste of the garden.

A Bit About Infused Waters

Here's an added extra about the latest Infused Waters that are hitting the food trends lately. With so much controversy surrounding energy drinks, sweeteners, fizzy drinks and health drinks that aren't really that "healthy", maybe we need some inspiration to welcome infused waters in to our lives?

Not everyone can face plain water, so a homemade, naturally flavored water is a great way to drink more and not compromise your hydro fitness. The benefit to this is that you can organize this ahead of time, leave water to infuse in the fridge and then help yourself to a naturally flavored drink, totally made up to suit your palate and taste, whenever you want. A collection of really pretty glasses and jugs are great accessories for these waters and can make them even more appealing. Imagine a glass jug filled with the most delicious raspberry and blueberry infused water, with ice, mint leaves and a juicy berries bobbing up and down. There will be a few less artificially flavored, expensive waters being purchased!

If you have a bit of a sweet tooth and find yourself with a dip in mood, a fruit infused water maybe also be able to curb your craving before you start hunting for a sugary snack. Infused waters are not just a brilliant way to stay hydrated, they are also a good way to lose weight. With only a few calories per glass, they will offer some guilt free sipping and a bit less time thinking "food".

Infused Waters are also very good for bloating and other digestive issues. Citrus infused water can help settle your stomach and have a calming effect on your body. A great replacement to a cup of coffee in the morning would be a tall glass of lemon infused water, which would set your digestive system up for the day.

There are some well-designed flasks on the market now that will allow you to pop a number of ingredients in to a central "core". You then fill the flask with water and leave to gently infuse whilst you go about your day. This is a great way to get a hydration takeaway that can be transported easily.

How about imagining some of these infused waters in your fridge, ready to quench your thirst? Would you be tempted to pass on the sweetened drinks and cordials? Welcome some natural hydration in to your life!

These waters all make approximately 1 liter of liquid (roughly 1/2 of your daily recommended intake). You can strain the drinks through a strainer if you like prior to serving, or leave them in.

Mint, Cucumber and Lime Vitality

Refreshment doesn't come much better than this. Mint and cucumber have such a "clean" flavor that you'll know you're getting their great anti-oxidant abilities as you sip on this drink. The lime adds a touch of sour that works so well.

Ingredients
- 1 large bunch of mint leaves
- 4 inch barrel of cucumber
- 2 limes
- 1 liter of water - filtered if liked

Instructions
1. Place water in a suitable jug/container.

2. Slice the cucumber in half and then cut in to semi circle disks

3. Slice 1 lime in to thin pieces. Juice the other lime.

4. Wash the mint and give it a bit of a "squeeze" to start releasing some of its flavor.

5. Add the lime juice and all of the ingredients to the water, give it a really good stir and place in the fridge for at least 1 hour.

Grapefruit and Rosemary Twining

If you haven't got a huge sweet tooth and yearn for something a little different, this is definitely worth stirring up. The grapefruit is a citrus fruit that will help combat bloating and digestive discomfort and blends well with the rosemary flavor.

Ingredients
- 3 sprigs of rosemary
- 1 grapefruit
- 1 liter of water

Instructions
1. Pour the water in to a suitable container or jug.

2. Wash the rosemary and give it a bit if a "scrunch" to release some of the flavor. Put in to the water.

3. Remove the skin from the grapefruit and cut in to segments. Add to the water.

4. Put the water with ingredients in to the fridge and leave to infuse for an hour. Give it a really good stir before it goes in to the fridge to get the flavors started.

Raspberry and Melon Infusion

Raspberries are full of ellagic acid that can assist in the prevention of cancer. They have the most glorious color to add to infused water. Either fresh, or frozen raspberries could be used for the recipe, but the riper, the slushier the better! The melon adds the sweetness to the raspberries that balances the flavor well.

Ingredients
- 2 handfuls of raspberries (frozen or fresh)
- ½ melon
- 1 liter of water – filtered if liked

Instructions
1. Pour the water in to a suitable container or jug.

2. Wash the raspberries and give them a little squash on a plate (so to catch the juices). Pour in to the water.

3. Cut the melon in to small pieces and add to the water.

4. Stir really well and place the container or jug in to the fridge for an hour to infuse.

Immune Booster

This is a refreshing, vitamin C packed infusion that delicately hydrates and gives you a great boost.

Ingredients
- 1 orange
- 1 lemon
- ½ mango
- 0.5 inch piece of ginger
- 1 liter of water – filtered if liked.

Instructions
1. Pour the water in to a container or jug.

2. Wash the lemon and orange and peel them. Cut the segments in to chunks.

3. Chop the mango in to bite size pieces.

4. Give the ginger a bit of scrape with a fork, to release some of the flavor.

5. Place the ingredients in to the jug or container, stir well and place in the fridge for at least an hour.

Detox Water

There are fruits that are known for their ability to provide anti-oxidant support to the body. With this infused water, a number of these fruits have been added to really enhance this hydration to work as a great detox assistance.

Ingredients
- 1 cup of blueberries
- 1 cup red grapes
- 1 apple
- ½ cup strawberries
- 1 orange
- 1 liter of water – filtered if liked

Instructions
1. Pour the water in to a suitable container or jug.

2. Wash the blueberries, grapes and strawberries. Give a few of them a bit of a squash to get the flavors releasing.

3. Wash the apple and cut in to thin slices.

4. Juice half the orange and cut the remaining orange in to thin slices.

5. Add the ingredients to the water, stir well and place in the fridge for at least one hour.

Passion Drink

Passion fruit has a really unique flavor that adds a bit of the "tropical" to your mouth. A great thirst quencher, this drink has added fruits that assist with lowering blood pressure.

Ingredients
- 2 passion fruits
- 2 kiwis
- 1 pomegranate
- 1 cup of cherries
- 1 liter of water – filtered if liked

Instructions
1. Pour the water in to a suitable container or jug.

2. Cut the passion fruit in half and scoop the seeds in to the water.

3. Peel the kiwis and slice. Add to the water.

4. Cut the pomegranate in half, tap and scoop the seeds out and then place ½ a cup of the seeds in to the water. Save the rest for another recipe.

5. Wash the cherries and remove the stones. Cut in half, squash a little on a plate and pour in to the water.

6. Stir really well and place the water in to the fridge for an hour at least.

Lemon, Ginger and Apple Infusion

This recipe calls for lemon verbena, which is delicate herb that has the most delicious lemon flavor. The addition of ginger and apple is a great twist that builds on a further level of flavor to be hydrated by.

Ingredients
- 1 large bunch of lemon verbena
- 1.5 inch piece of fresh ginger root
- 1 apple
- 1 liter of water - filtered if liked.

Instructions
1. Pour the water in to a suitable container or jug.

2. Wash the lemon verbena, give it a bit of a "scrunch" and place in to the water.

3. Wash the ginger root and give it a rough peel with a spoon. Slice in to pieces and add to the water.

4. Wash the apple, core and slice in to thin pieces. Add to the water.

5. Stir really well and place the water in to the fridge for at least an hour.

Peach and Sage Herbal Hydration

This is an unusual combination that works well. You could create some of your own unusual flavors to try? This can give you another reason to drink more as you can count on your curiosity asking "now, what DOES that taste like?" This can sometimes shout a bit louder than a nagging mildly, dehydrated body.

Ingredients
- 3 peaches - ripe
- 1 large bunch of sage
- 1 liter of water – filtered if liked.

Instructions
1. Pour the water in to a suitable container or jug.

2. Wash the peaches and slice thinly, discarding the stones. Reserve a handful of pieces and add the rest to the water.

3. On a plate, squash the reserved peach pieces to start releasing flavor. Tip contents from the plate in the water.

4. Wash the sage and "scrunch" a little in your hands before adding to the water.

5. Give the water a really good stir and place in the fridge for at least an hour.

Watermelon and Mint Refresher

Watermelon has a light, delicate freshness that is a great addition to a hydrating drink. With a good helping of vitamins A, B6 and C, it is known to provide some good nutrition, plus a great hydrating factor being made up mainly of water. Make sure you eat these pieces of fruit too for the most effective hydration.

Ingredients
- ½ a medium sized watermelon
- 1 medium bunch of fresh mint
- 1 liter of water, filtered if liked

Instructions
1. Pour the water in to a suitable container or jug.
2. Cut the watermelon in to bite size pieces and place in the water.
3. Wash the mint and give it a bit of a "squeeze" to start releasing some minty flavor.
4. Add to the water too and give it a really good stir.
5. Place the water in to the fridge and leave to infuse for at least one hour.

Basil, Mint and Lemon Squeeze

Basil has a quite a strong aroma and really lends itself well to a refreshing drink. It acts as an anti-inflammatory agent and can be useful with reducing stress. It's a herb that is sometimes added to sweets and desserts so its not as savory as some. Go on, give this one a go, just to satisfy the curiosity!

Ingredients
- 1 medium bunch of basil
- 1 small bunch of mint
- 2 lemons
- 1 liter of water – filtered if liked

Instructions
1. Pour the water in to a suitable container or jug.

2. Wash the basil, mint and lemons.

3. "Scrunch" both the basil and mint, to start releasing their flavor and add to the water.

4. Squeeze the juice from one of the lemons and pour in to the water.

5. With the other lemon, slice finely and add to the water.

6. Give the water a really good stir and place in the fridge for at least an hour.

Chia Strawberry Fruit Cup

Chia is already well known for its ability to add protein and good omega 3 fat to a diet. The Mexican's have long used a drink called Chia Fresca, which is made up of chia seeds, a sweetener, water and lemon or lime. It's an excellent way to not just promote better hydration but it also provides a huge blast of energy. It is a different texture than plain water, due to its nature of turning in to thickened jelly balls, which are a delight to many! Don't leave this one sitting for longer than a few hours though, unless you like it really thick!

Ingredients
- 1 cup of strawberries
- 2 lemons
- 1 tbsp chia seeds
- 1 liter of water – filtered if liked

Instructions
1. Pour the water in to a suitable container or jug.

2. Wash and hull the strawberries. Roughly chop them on a plate, to catch any juice and tip in to the water.

3. Juice one of the lemons and pour in to the water. Slice the other lemon thinly and place in to the water.

4. Stir in the chia seeds and give it all a good mix. Place in the fridge for at least an hour and see what develops!

Chia Mint Cup

This is another adaption of the Mexican Drink, Chia Fresca. Mint imparts a healthy freshness to this drink. A settling, hydrating and digestive support, this is a drink to really help relax a stressed stomach.

Ingredients
- 1 large bunch of mint leaves
- 1 lime
- 1 tbsp of chia seeds
- 1 liter of water – filtered if liked

Instructions
1. Pour the water in to a suitable container or jug.

2. Wash the mint leaves and "scrunch" them up a little. Place in the jug.

3. Wash the lime and slice in to the thin pieces. Add to the water.

4. Stir in the chia seeds and give it all a good mix.

5. Place the water in to the fridge for at least an hour.

Rose, Strawberry and Lemon Cooler

Rose is quite a delicate flavor but can go so well with some of the sweet flavors from the garden. Rose and strawberry seem to have a great taste together and both add some "girlie color" to a hydrating drink.

Ingredients
- 1 cup of strawberries
- 1 tbsp dried rose petals
- 2 lemons
- 1 liter of water – filtered if liked

Instructions
1. Pour the water in to a suitable container or jug.

2. Wash the hull the strawberries. Slice in to thin pieces and add to the water.

3. Wash the lemons. Juice one of them, adding to the water. Slice the other one in to thin slices and add to the water.

4. Tip in the rose petals and give it all a really good stir.

5. This could benefit for being refrigerated for at least 2 hours to get some deeper flavor from the roses.

Cinnamon and Apple Water

This is a flavor combination already tried and tested over the years and certainly works well. Try to find the Ceylon Cinnamon for this as it's really the king of cinnamon and will provide you with the best health benefits. Choose a really sweet apple variety to help balance the pungent aromatic from the cinnamon.

Ingredients
- 2 tsp ground cinnamon (Ceylon if you can find it)
- 1 cinnamon stick
- 3 apples
- ½ lemon
- 1 liter of water – filtered if liked

Instructions
1. Pour the water in to a suitable container or jug.

2. Wash and core the apples.

3. Slice the apples thinly, crushing a few on a plate to catch any juices.

4. Add to the water.

5. Slice the lemon thinly and add to the water.

6. Stir in the cinnamon. Break the cinnamon stick in half and add to the water too.

7. Give the water a really good mix. This infusion would be best to develop in the fridge over night, or for at least 2 hours.

Pomegranate, Lime and Ginger Infusion

Pomegranate, when ripe, is a sweet Middle Eastern fruit that claims to help reduce the risk of heart disease, reduce blood pressure and reduce inflammation. You may want to hydrate with this drink and consume these lovely little seeds as you go!

Ingredients
- 1 pomegranate
- 2 limes
- 1.5 inch piece root ginger
- 1 liter of water – filtered if liked.

Instructions
1. Pour the water in to a suitable container or jug.

2. Half the pomegranate, give it a tap and remove the seeds. Add them to the water.

3. Wash the limes.

4. Juice one of the limes and slice the other in to thin pieces.

5. Roughly peel the ginger and slice in to thin pieces.

6. Add the ginger and lime to the water and pomegranate.

7. Give the water a really good stir. This water infusion may be best left to develop for at least 2 hours.

Oregano, Blueberry and Lime Refresher

Blueberries are known for their anti-oxidant providing abilities and they are wonderfully sweet. Add the addition of spicy herb and a lime twist, and you have a hydrating drink that could almost be given the label "super".

Ingredients
- 2 cups of blueberries
- 2 limes
- 1 medium bunch of fresh oregano
- 1 liter of water – filtered if liked

Instructions
1. Pour the water in to a suitable container or jug.

2. Wash the blueberries and limes.

3. Add the blueberries to the water, squashing a third of them on to a plate beforehand, and catching any juice to add too.

4. Juice one of the limes and add the juice to the water. Slice the other lime in to thin pieces.

5. Wash the oregano and give it a bit of a "squeeze" to start releasing some of it's flavor.

6. Add the herbs to the water and mix really well. Leave in the fridge for at least an hour before serving.

Coconut and Peach Infusion

This water infusion uses coconut water as a base. Although containing sugar, it is well studied and proven to help improve hydration. After a workout, it could be a good base to add to your infusions and always better than added sugar sports drinks.

Ingredients
- 1 cup of coconut water
- 1 peaches
- Handful of ice

Instructions
1. Pour water in to a suitable container or jug.

2. Wash the peach and remove the stone. Chop in to small pieces, squashing a few of the pieces to start the flavor going and add to the water.

3. Store in the fridge for 2-3 hours. Serve with a good handful of ice.

Coconut Water Raspberry Lemon Mix

This is another good post workout drink, using coconut water. There are a number of flavored coconut waters on the market, but why spend the extra on them when they are this easy to make!

Ingredients
- 1 cup of coconut water
- 1 cup of fresh or frozen raspberries
- 8 lemon verbena leaves
- Handful of ice

Instructions
1. Pour the water in to a suitable container or jug

2. Wash the raspberries and give them a bit of squeeze on a plate. Pour the raspberries and any juices in to the water.

3. Wash the lemon verbena leaves and "scrunch" them up a bit to start releasing the flavor. Add to the water

4. Place the water in the fridge for 2-3 hours.

5. Serve with a big handful of ice.

Pineapple and Mint Cup

Vitamin C and Beta-carotene are found in the sweet flesh of the pineapple so this a great immune boosting, hydrating drink. Try to ensure the pineapple is ripe so this infusion has a lovely sweetness to work with the mint.

Ingredients
- 2 cups of chopped pineapple pieces (can be from a can, but make sure it's one that was not in "syrup")
- 1 medium bunch of mint leaves
- 1 liter of water – filtered if liked

Instructions
1. Pour the water in to a suitable container or jug.

2. Tip the pineapple pieces in to the water and give it a really good mix. Try squashing a few pieces with a fork to get that pineapple flavor seeping out.

3. Wash the mint leaves and roughly "squeeze". Add to the water.

4. Stir the water really well and place in the fridge for at least 1 hour.

Orange and Tarragon Refreshment

Tarragon is quite a strong flavor so don't add too much. However, it's a rich source of Vitamin A and minerals such as magnesium, iron and zinc so it makes a great functional and hydrating infusion. The orange balances the flavor well to produce quite a unique taste.

Ingredients
- 2 oranges
- 1 medium bunch of tarragon
- 1 liter of water – filtered if liked

Instructions
1. Pour the water in to a suitable container or jug.

2. Wash the oranges. Juice one of the oranges and add to the water. Slice the other thinly and add to the water too.

3. Wash the tarragon well and give it a bit of a "squeeze" to release some of its flavor.

4. Add the tarragon to the water and oranges. Give it a really good stir and place in the fridge for an hour to let the flavor develop.

Thirst Quencher

This infused water is pure refreshment, light flavors with a touch of sweetness. Replacing lost fluid through exercise and sweat really is important after a work out, so try this one. Leave it in the fridge and have it handy to re-hydrate.

Ingredients
- 1 cup of watermelon
- 1 peach
- ½ cup raspberries
- ½ orange
- 1 sprig of lemon thyme
- 1 liter of water – filtered if liked

Instructions
1. Cut the water melon in to bite size pieces.

2. Wash the peach, half and remove the stone. Cut in slices

3. Wash the raspberries and on a plate, give them a bit of a squash.

4. Give the thyme a good "scrunch".

5. Pour the water in to a suitable container or jug. Add all of the ingredients to the water and leave in the fridge for 1-2 hours at least to infuse.

6. Serve in a tall glass with lots of crushed ice and a straw.

Hibiscus, Lemon and Cherry Sour

Hibiscus has quite a floral sourness that blends well with the lemon in this recipe. Hibiscus is known to help digestion, high blood pressure and depression. Try to find some really ripe cherries for this as the color will be a glorious purple hue that will look so appealing. Orange segments and crushed ice are the perfect accompaniment.

Ingredients
- 1 tsp dried hibiscus flowers
- 1 cup ripe cherries
- 1 lemon
- 1 orange
- 1 liter of water – filtered if liked
- Crushed Ice to Serve

Instructions
1. Pour the water in to a suitable container or jug.

2. Rub the dried hibiscus flowers and place in the water

3. Stone the cherries and cut them in half. On a plate, to save any juices, give half of them a bit of a squeeze. Pour in to the water.

4. Juice half the lemon and cut the other half in to thin slices.

5. Juice half the orange and cut the other half in to thin slices.

6. Add the juices and the lemon and orange slices to the water and store in the fridge for at least 2-3 hours to let the hibiscus petals re-hydrate and infuse their benefits in to the water.

7. Enjoy ice cold.

Pink Lemon Aid

A simple infusion can sometimes be the most effective. Raspberry, blackcurrants and lemon add a shot of Vitamin C to this rehydrating tonic, with the added bonus of looking pretty too. The stevia leaves are a great way to add a bit of natural sweetness to this sour infused water and it looks really appealing when serving. Try and grow some stevia in a kitchen pot at home, as it can be a really versatile sweetener to add to any dishes. You could dry some leaves in a warm spot so you can crumble them in to some recipes, instead of relying on the expensive powders.

Ingredients
- 1 lemon
- 1 cup of raspberries
- ½ cup of blackcurrants
- A small bunch of stevia leaves
- 1 liter of water – filtered if liked.

Instructions
1. Pour the water in to a suitable container or jug.

2. Wash the raspberries. Squash a few on a plate, and pour them and then other raspberries in to the water.

3. Wash the blackcurrants and squash a few of these in the same way before adding to the water.

4. Half the lemon and juice it. With the other half, slice thinly. Add the slices and juice to the water.

5. Add the stevia leaves to the water and place the container in the fridge for 1-2 hours to infuse.

6. Serve with crushed ice.

Conclusion

It can be so easy to fall in to the trap of being tempted by sugar-added drinks to quench a thirst; especially when you are out and about. Have you ever noticed that many stores have brightly colored, "stand out" displays of sports drinks, fizzy drinks and juices with added sugars? They tend to be put on shelves at eye level and when you're in a rush and need to grab a drink, it's sometimes the easiest thing to buy. What's the alternative; a bottle of plain water? Not any more!

As with any healthy eating plan, or particular diet you are following, it does require an element of pre-planning. If you want to embrace a wonderful new, energized body through hydration, you will need a little pre-thought with this too. It can be so easy though! If you are preparing a salad or fruit dish, cut a little extra. Increase the herbs you use in your cooking and prepare a few more when you're preparing. Fill a couple of bottles of water up for the fridge and pop those extra ingredients in to them as you're chopping. Easy.

*Before you embark on a whirlwind of blending, whizzing, steeping, juicing and infusing in your kitchen, it's worth noting that fruits and nut waters and milks, all do contain high levels of sugar. Try to choose herb based and vegetable based drinks a little more than the fruity ones, as they won't impact your blood sugar levels quite as much.

Finally, it may be worth taking a moment to think about the benefits of using these recipes and being fully hydrated. Your body would thank you for not "forgetting" it again in the future! So here goes-

The Benefits of Alkaline Vegan Drinks aka Hydro-Fit Hydration

- Reaching for a natural drink when you feel hungry may be a good way to control weight, as many of us mistaken the signs of thirst, as hunger.
- Your body will feel more energized as it is able to flush out toxins more quickly.
- It's easy to stay on an eating plan or dietary lifestyle, as you are able to tailor make drinks to suit you.
- Your mental health will improve with a well-hydrated body, allowing you to think better and perform better.
- If you are someone who struggles to consume the recommended 5 portions of fruit or vegetable a day, you can easily achieve this in some delicious smoothies and juices.
- Your skin will be clearer and feel smoother.
- Your cardio-vascular health will be optimized.
- Good hydration supports the work your joints and muscles need to do.
- It helps control your body temperature
- It can assist a weight loss plan where you can still stay well nourished by using nutrient packed, filling smoothies as meal replacements.
- You can exercise for longer, be stronger and prevents injuries.

Hydration is so important to our wellbeing and these recipes have hopefully created some inspiration to help you give some more thought to your liquid diet than you perhaps do currently.

So get set, get energized and feel hydro-fit!

Free eBook & Inspirational Vegan Friendly Newsletter

Before you go, I would like to offer you a free, complimentary eBook + free newsletter that goes with it (with even more information about vegan recipes).

We are in this together!

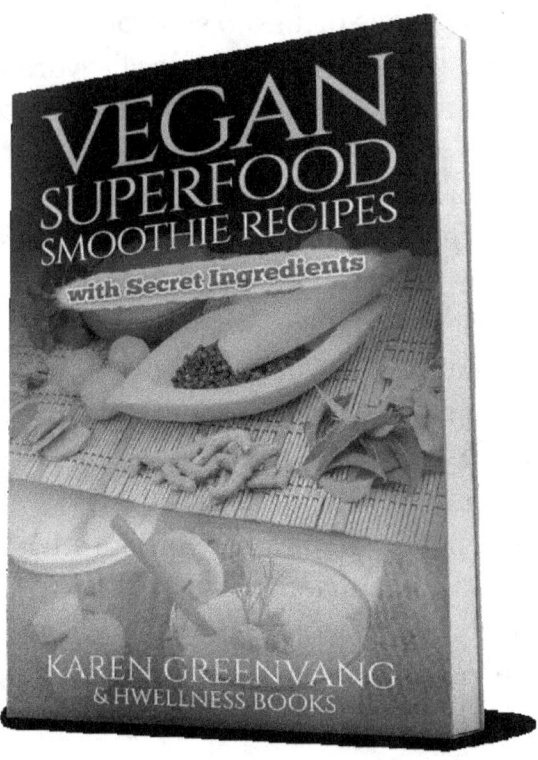

Simply visit:

www.holisticwellnessbooks.com/vegan to grab your free copy by joining my newsletter.

In case you happen to have any technical problems- email me at:
karen@holisticwellnessbooks.com and I will be happy to help! Thank you again for taking an interest in my work. I hope you will enjoy this free bonus!

www.ingramcontent.com/pod-product-compliance
Lightning Source LLC
Chambersburg PA
CBHW071622080526
44588CB00010B/1231